Ted Freeman

and the Battle for the Injured Brain

A case history of professional prejudice

Peter McCullagh

Ted Freeman

and the Battle for the Injured Brain

A case history of professional prejudice

Peter McCullagh

Australian National University

E PRESS

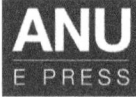

ANU E PRESS

Published by ANU E Press
The Australian National University
Canberra ACT 0200, Australia
Email: anuepress@anu.edu.au
This title is also available online at http://epress.anu.edu.au

National Library of Australia Cataloguing-in-Publication entry

Author: McCullagh, Peter.

Title: Ted Freeman and the battle for the injured brain : a case history of professional
             prejudice / Peter McCullagh.

ISBN: 9781922144317 (paperback) 9781922144324 (ebook)

Subjects: Freeman, E. A. (Edward Alan)
             Coma--Treatment.
             Coma--Patients--Rehabilitation.
             Brain damage--Treatment.
             Brain damage--Patients--Rehabilitation.
             Brain--Treatment.
             Brain--Wounds and injuries--Rehabilitation.

Dewey Number: 616.8046

Cover photograph courtesy of Dorothy Freeman.

Cover design and layout by ANU E Press

Contents

Acknowledgments

This book is intended to represent, in a small way, an acknowledgment of the achievements of people with brain injury and their families. Some of those who sought assistance from Dr Ted Freeman after the Australian healthcare system effectively discarded them are described in the book. They are intended to be a representative selection of the people who sought his help over two decades. Some achieved remarkable results; others were much less spectacular. Some failed to improve; others died suddenly and unexpectedly, often after making good progress. An unknown number of young victims of motor vehicle accidents lacked a family able to intervene on their behalf and may spend up to five decades in aged-care institutions.

Traumatic brain injury dominated the life of Ted Freeman for several decades. This book would not exist had he not documented his experiences with patients, their families and his professional colleagues. He generously provided access to everything that he had saved and written.

During the period of compilation of the manuscript, I have received notable help and encouragement from people at The Australian National University. Professor Marian Sawer and her committee have provided many suggestions that, when incorporated in the text, have greatly improved it. A member of the committee, Dr Gwen Gray, made an extraordinary contribution to the book, going through it sentence by sentence and suggesting modifications and posing questions to be answered in the revised text. I am very heavily in her debt. When it came to presenting the manuscript in a form suitable for review, my fairly primitive word-processing skills received unstinting help from Alison Plumb. I am most appreciative of her assistance in aiming for a presentable manuscript.

Peter McCullagh

Acronyms

AAN	Australian Association of Neurologists
ACBIC	Australian Centre for Brain Injured Children
AMA	Australian Medical Association
BIOS	Brain Injury Outcome Study
BIRP	Brain Injury Rehabilitation Program
BITC	Brain Injury Therapy Centre
FRCSE	Fellowship of the Royal College of Surgeons of Edinburgh
GCS	Glasgow Coma Scale
GIO	Government Insurance Office (NSW)
IAHP	Institutes for the Achievement of Human Potential
IASTBI	International Association for the Study of Traumatic Brain Injury
MCS	minimally conscious state
NBIF	National Brain Injury Foundation
NDIS	National Disability Insurance Scheme
NHIF	National Head Injury Foundation (US)
NHMRC	National Health and Medical Research Council
PVS	persistent vegetative state
SMART	sensory modality assessment rehabilitation and treatment
TBI	traumatic brain injury
WHO	World Health Organisation

Preface

All truth passes through three stages
First it is ridiculed
Second it is violently opposed
Third it is accepted as being self-evident.

— Arthur Schopenhauer (1788–1860)

As its title implies, this book tells the story of an individual and his career commitment. It also describes the antagonistic response of some of his colleagues.

The individual, Dr Ted Freeman, developed a compelling interest, which he pursued at considerable personal cost, in the potential for long-term rehabilitation of people who had sustained an acquired brain injury. The people whom he wished to assist had, invariably, been excluded from mainstream medicine on the grounds that they were 'unsuitable for rehabilitation'. Freeman's response to their exclusion followed a rather logical course—namely, designing rehabilitation programs that were predominantly dependent upon families, friends and volunteers. This involvement of non-medical personnel in rehabilitation undoubtedly fuelled some of the antagonism that he experienced.

Redirecting his career pathway, Freeman pursued his interest in attempting rehabilitation of people with brain injuries for whom conventional approaches had nothing to offer. He studied the limited information on repair processes after brain injury available in the medical literature in the early 1980s. Taking account of this, he formulated some hypotheses and proceeded to apply the implications drawn from these in his clinical practice.

In 1988, I was contacted on behalf of a group of people who were in the process of establishing the National Brain Injury Foundation (NBIF) and were keen to have a medically qualified person as a board member. Some of these people had personal experience of brain injury and its aftermath. Shortly after this, I first met Ted Freeman. The NBIF had been conceived as a community-based organisation the goal of which was to provide whatever form of practical assistance could help people with acquired brain injury. Such assistance was usually given by working through patients' families. Ted Freeman had come to the aid of many of the families who became NBIF members and, throughout the 1980s and 1990s, he had frequent contact with the Foundation. Until his retirement in 2000, the NBIF sought to support the man and his work. On some occasions, when he visited patients in Canberra, I had the opportunity to sit in on his meetings with them and their families and found his approach to be as described below.

As president of the Foundation for 12 years, I had regular contact with Ted and was aware that he had collated an account of his experiences with a view to publication. In order to facilitate this, he retained copies of relevant letters and other documents. All of the items to which reference is made in this account are held by him. When he decided not to proceed with writing an account of his experiences, I offered to assist him with the project. In the event, he declined joint authorship and the result has been a book about him rather than one written collaboratively with him.

In reviewing the manuscript, as it neared completion, Ted wrote that his concern had been and remained

> *the systemic failure of the medical profession in both diagnosis and treatment of severe brain injury. My position is that I was a vehicle to bring the failures of that system to public and professional notice—nothing more.*

He said to me:

> *I see that still to be the substance and challenge of the book you have written and that you also are a vehicle of disclosure.*

In the course of preparation of the manuscript, I have extracted much information from his account, supplemented by frequent discussion with him, but I have also taken the opportunity to draw what I consider to be some more widely applicable inferences about issues raised by his experiences.

When using Ted's material, I have chosen to present different aspects of brain injury together with his responses to these in separate chapters rather than following his original chronological account. This has entailed separation into two parallel narratives dealing with the evolution of his practice and with the concurrent events that impacted upon that evolution. This has some distinct advantages and some drawbacks. A significant advantage is that it becomes possible to discuss any specific aspect, such as his impact on management of comatose patients in Chapter 4, as a single entity rather than returning to it and discussing it piecemeal on several occasions. Most helpfully, it facilitates consideration of wider implications of an event, such as the clinical trial in Chapter 6, without having to interrupt a chronological account.

A drawback of moving away from a chronological account is that it becomes necessary at some places in the text to recapitulate detail from an earlier chapter if that detail is essential to an explanation of why particular events occurred. Chapter 5, which deals with the evolution of Freeman's practices, insofar as they relate to patients who have regained consciousness after a brain injury, spans a period of more than 15 years. During this time, Freeman's base moved from one of Sydney's largest public hospitals to a purpose-modified centre and then to a caravan travelling around New South Wales. A full account of the events occasioning the three moves will be provided in Chapters 6 and 7 but the aggregation within a single chapter of Freeman's activities over the three stages is intended to shed light on the manner in which evolution of his practice was influenced by external events.

Introduction

The work of Ted Freeman and the local medical profession's response to it raise several critical issues that have ongoing relevance for Australian health consumers and health policymakers alike. The first is the capacity of the health system to respond appropriately to catastrophic disablement. Until the 1980s, at least, the conditions in which many people with severe disabilities were kept shocked most outside observers. Today, awareness is higher and more resources have been allocated, but long-term care institutions remain the subject of myriad complaints.

Another worrying issue that his story raises is the closure of some medical minds and the isolation of the Australian medical fraternity from the latest overseas developments in treatment. Dr Freeman was widely ostracised by colleagues who appear to have been unaware of the cutting-edge ideas and practices that were emerging in other countries where his work was highly respected. Since the 1980s, Freeman's hypotheses that the brain is plastic and has considerable capacity to repair itself have been validated by scientific observations and are now universally accepted. Australian health consumers might well ask whether mechanisms are in place to prevent a recurrence of such a travesty.

The issue of what constitutes evidence-based medicine is as relevant today as it was 30 years ago. In its bid to ensure legitimacy, medical practice has emphasised the scientific basis of that practice; however, a quick survey reveals that many practices have been introduced on the basis of empirical evidence long before modes of operation were understood. The reality that there was no scientific basis, in the 1980s, for the commonly accepted approach to the management of people with injured brains is a case in point.

The relationship between scientific hypothesis, including its validation, and empirical observation in developing potentially innovative medical therapies is a central issue in the Freeman story. Demonstration that a specific therapy can benefit a group of patients, without imposing a contingent risk, is not synonymous with an equally confident demonstration of how that therapy is actually achieving its goal.

The introduction of penicillin into clinical practice may be the best-known example of the reality that demonstration of clinical efficacy and safety is a question distinct from that of how an innovative therapy is actually achieving its results. Clinical proof of the value of this antibiotic was established by Howard Florey in the early 1940s and was sufficiently convincing that its use in the North African theatre of World War II was expedited. Understanding of the mechanism of action of penicillin, however, had to await the crystallographic studies of its structure by Dorothy Crowfoot Hodgkin two decades later. This gap was reflected in the two decades separating the awarding of Nobel prizes to Florey (Medicine or Physiology, 1945) and Hodgkin (Chemistry, 1964).

In other instances, a therapeutic advance has been successfully introduced underpinned by a hypothesis of its mechanism of action that has subsequently been invalidated by further research with the result that this hypothesis has been discarded. Nevertheless, clinical efficacy, accompanied by safety, has ensured the continued use of the therapy, notwithstanding the abandonment of the theory that originally led to its development.

In 2013, successful new therapies are increasingly being produced by synthesis of molecules the detailed structure of which may be predicted in advance to act on highly specific cellular receptors in the human body. These receptors have, in their turn, been shown previously to be critical in disease development. On this basis, it is easy to assume, quite incorrectly, that empiricism had no place in twentieth-century medicine. Despite the elegance of therapeutic approaches developed by molecular strategies, it is unlikely that anything approaching the full range of human diseases will be so well understood in the foreseeable future. Acquired brain injury and the mechanisms responsible for recovery, at least at the molecular level, are likely to elude such precise understanding. The experience to date, including that of Freeman, implies that interventions that are much more basic and which defy precise measurement, such as human interactions, may continue to have more to offer.

Acquired brain injury and, more specifically, the potential for recovery from it, was very poorly understood at the time Freeman became interested in the subject. His initiatives, to be discussed in this book, were based on the limited understanding of normal function and capacity for repair following injury in the human brain available at the time. Understanding of these events, although it has advanced since the early 1980s, remains massively incomplete today. The truism that 'if the human brain was sufficiently simple that we could understand it using our own brains, we wouldn't have the ability to do so' remains substantially valid.

Freeman's hypotheses about which approaches might facilitate recovery of the injured brain were substantially based on the body of information that had been published to that time, with one notable exception—namely, that of the existence of neuroplasticity. Much of this information is likely to have been wide of the mark. One basis for opposition to his proposals by colleagues was undoubtedly that they conflated assessment of his hypotheses with his clinical outcomes. To the extent that some of his hypotheses could be associated with claims by others, which may have been of dubious validity, opposition was fuelled.

Reinforcing the opposition to Freeman engendered by scepticism about his theories, divorced from the question of whether the clinical outcomes of people who had participated in programs designed by him were successful, was an attitude that can only be categorised as therapeutic nihilism. Details of this will be given in a later chapter but its basis may be summarised here. The prevailing mind-set (I do not consider that an unduly denigratory term in this context) among medical professionals at the time when Freeman set out to attempt rehabilitation of people with severe brain injury held that any recovery could only occur as a result of a natural process. Furthermore, it held that the speed and extent of any recovery would not be affected by medical intervention. As succinctly expressed at the time, the medical attendants were no more than spectators during the return of consciousness. This firmly held opinion, which Freeman would not accept, was buttressed by the scientific conviction that new neurons could not be formed after birth in the human brain.

Controversially at the time, Freeman hypothesised that brain repair was possible, whether by the production of new cells, by the assumption of new responsibilities by existing networks of cells or by other, unanticipated mechanisms. These processes fell into the description, disparaged at the time, of 'neuroplasticity'. Freeman's records indicate that he was actively promoting the concept of plasticity as a contributor to functional recovery in the early 1980s. The term 'neuroplasticity' and the concept underlying it are now universally accepted. One type of observation facilitating this acceptance has been the repeated demonstration of the formation of new neurons. Whether, and to what extent, the generation of new neurons contributed to the recoveries that ensued among many of Freeman's patients is unknown but, by analogy with the history of the introduction of penicillin into practice already referred to, that is not a valid reason to preclude clinical application.

Background

The outlook for a patient with acquired brain injury in 1980 was a reflection of rapid progress in one field of medical practice, unaccompanied by comparable progress in associated fields. Advances in intensive care, and in radiological technology capable of very accurately localising injury within the brain in anticipation of emergency neurosurgery, permitted the survival beyond the acute stage of many patients with traumatic injury who would not formerly have done so. A majority of these patients were young persons involved in motor vehicle accidents. By the time that their need for intensive care had been replaced by a need for rehabilitation, some of these people would not have regained consciousness and, of those who had done so, many remained very severely disabled.

Existing rehabilitation services were not usually equipped to meet the needs of patients who remained severely disabled by brain injury when they were discharged from an intensive care unit. Furthermore, because of budgetary constraints, rehabilitation services commonly imposed minimal entry standards, which were unattainable by these patients. Consequently, patients who had sustained severe traumatic brain injuries in the first three decades of life, along with those who had sustained other types of severe neurological impairment, were frequently destined for admission to aged-care facilities at an early stage, sometimes within a few weeks of the event occasioning their injury. This major deficiency in provision of continuity of health care required that patients conformed to the established system or were excluded from it. An alternative—namely, that of introducing systemic flexibility, for example, in the form of slow-stream rehabilitation strategies—was not accepted, at least in Australia, in the 1980s. Having witnessed the fate of young adults consigned to nursing homes for the remainder of their lives (which most of his colleagues are unlikely to have done), Freeman felt compelled to intervene on their behalf. Many of the patients whom Freeman attended under the auspices of the National Brain Injury Foundation conformed to this description.

Medical tribalism (or the dominance of the curative medical model)

The disconnection between the acute care provided to patients with an acquired brain injury and that available in the longer term serves to highlight a second general issue exposed by Freeman's experience—namely, the consequences for a patient of medical tribalism. This was manifest in segmentation of different aspects of a patient's care and accompanied by an emphasis on cure at the expense of care. An example of this, discussed below, was the setting of fixed time boundaries between the care to be provided by different medical specialties, irrespective of an individual patient's progress along the recovery path. Patient transfer from one speciality to another was likely to follow the systemic rules rather than the specific patient's needs. These demarcation issues came to the fore in the course of trialling Freeman's practices in a hospital setting. Tribalism certainly came to the fore in the personal hostility directed towards Freeman by some of his medical colleagues. Being neither a neurologist nor an accredited rehabilitation specialist, he could not be taken seriously, it was suggested.

Before considering the nature of the issues raised in the course of attempts to trial Freeman's ideas, another source of antagonism towards him should be noted. An approach that he commonly adopted may be categorised as 'domiciliary rehabilitation'. This entailed the conduct of rehabilitation measures in the patient's home. Primary participants in such programs were family members, frequently assisted by large groups of volunteers. Not only did family members undertake procedures with their patient but also, not unnaturally, they often made observations. Freeman invariably took account of family observations, a practice with which some colleagues strongly disagreed. Moreover, the shifting of responsibility for rehabilitation from healthcare professionals to laypersons tended to generate hostility among healthcare professionals.

The basis cited by many practitioners for disparaging the reports from family members ranged across issues such as their lack of training and the risk that they would see what they hoped to see. Freeman's emphatic response to these objections was that he found family members to be accurate observers. It was also relevant that they had 24/7 access to patients rather than a few minutes in the course of a ward round. As discussed later, inconsistency in patient responsiveness is a characteristic feature during the early stages of regaining consciousness after brain injury. Several decades after Freeman stressed this inconsistency in responsiveness, some objective validation of it is now available.

The issue of formally showing whether Freeman's proposals for rehabilitation after severe brain injury, especially when followed by prolonged unconsciousness, were actually successful was very significant. As mentioned already, there was some tendency for this question to be intertwined with the question of whether Freeman's explanation of the responsible mechanism(s) was correct. As suggested above, the question of success should be separated from that of its mechanism.

A strong case can be made that the methodology that it was sought to apply to testing the success or otherwise of Freeman's rehabilitation strategies— namely, a double-blind randomised control trial—was utterly inappropriate in that situation. This point is examined in some detail in Chapter 6. Even the most sophisticated, 'state-of-the-art' technology may be rendered useless, and sometimes dangerously misguided, when applied in circumstances for which it is unsuited. Whilst such trials can be an essential aid in the evaluation of many new pharmaceutical agents and surgical procedures, it is not feasible to conduct them, nor will they provide any information of value, when applied to studies of the effect of intervention by family members on an unconscious patient. One size, most emphatically, does not fit all.

The deferral of this account until the second decade of the new century has provided the opportunity to revisit some of Freeman's practices in the light of an accumulating body of information gained by the application of novel imaging technology to patients who have been diagnosed as comatose. As a result, it can be confirmed that some of the clinical procedures that Freeman advocated and applied can actually initiate and influence brain activity in these people.

Recalling the caveat, already expressed, that there can be considerable value in observations even if their meaning is not fully understood, some reservations legitimately remain about the meaning of observations of electrical activity demonstrable in the brain. Whether a specific form of activity represents the actual mechanistic correlate of consciousness, rather than being an epiphenomenon, closely linked to but separate from that correlate, is probably unknowable and more likely to be a question for metaphysics than for medicine. Nevertheless, such observations offer much for improving the lot of individuals who have been incorrectly diagnosed as clinically unconscious.

There are two topics underlying the story of Freeman's battle, already dealt with in earlier publications, the details of which have not been introduced into this account. Whilst Freeman's philosophy relating to rehabilitation following brain injury and its practical application are frequently referred to, anyone seeking a comprehensive practical account is referred to his two handbooks on this subject.[1] Many of the patients who benefited from Freeman's advice, probably a majority, had been dismissed by others as 'vegetative'. This term was frequently inaccurate and invariably pejorative. I have refrained from any examination of the concept of vegetative states in this text but have previously pursued this subject in some depth.[2]

Three decades of achievement and controversy

Ted Freeman has had an interesting career, notable for its contrasts. Having left school, he worked as a barrow boy in the Sydney Markets but, 20 years later, was admitted as a Fellow of the Royal College of Surgeons of Edinburgh. While caring, as a general practitioner, for people whose lives had been disrupted by traumatic brain injury, his daily observations led him to propose major changes in attitudes towards their disabilities, and consequent modifications in their management. As a result of his achievements, he was to receive considerable international recognition. Notwithstanding that recognition, he was shunned by some of his Australian colleagues. He was defamed under parliamentary privilege, but went on to be recognised for his contributions to medicine in the Order of Australia awards.

In retrospect, most achievements may be traced, at least partially, to the experiences of the individual responsible for them. Chapter 1 contains Ted

---

1   Edward Freeman (1987) *The Catastrophe of Coma—A Way Back*. David Bateman, Buderim, Qld. (Available free online from the National Brain Injury Foundation: <http://nbif.org.au>); Edward Freeman (1998) *Brain Injury and Stroke—A Handbook to Recovery*. Hale & Iremonger, Sydney.
2   Peter McCullagh (2004) *Conscious in a Vegetative State? A Critique of the PVS Concept. Volume 23, International Library of Ethics, Law and the New Medicine*. Kluwer Academic Publishers, Dordrecht.

Freeman's account of some formative experiences. The personal experience of being unable to communicate following Freeman's inadvertent isolation after a hospital admission with meningitis afforded him an insight into the predicament of many individuals with brain injuries that was to stay with him. A chance observation of communication between a child with cerebral palsy and its mother, although that communication remained inaccessible to others, aroused his interest in the possibility of retention of undetected abilities in people with severe brain injury. As a response to these incidents, Freeman redirected his career, deliberately seeking to discover all that he could about the impact of brain injury on patients and their families. That concern led him to embark, in the first instance, on visits to relevant clinics overseas and then into related employment in Australia.

When he proposed and implemented substantial changes from existing practice, Freeman was warned by some of his colleagues, and unreservedly criticised by others. The declared basis for criticism was that the scientific backgrounds of some of the therapists from whom he sought to learn were regarded as suspect.

My reading of his own account of these events is that he was overwhelmingly influenced, primarily, by the care and concern for their patients manifest by those therapists. The contrast was indeed considerable when placed alongside his observations of attitudes prevalent in some Australian facilities towards those severely disabled by a variety of conditions including brain injury. In the absence of any accepted alternatives in mainstream medical practice, he was captured by the challenge of attempting to help, even in the most desperate situations.

Students are taught at an early stage in medical school that a good practitioner learns from his patients, an experience that Freeman has repeatedly recounted. That being so, it is natural that any account of the philosophy and practices that he refined over the course of his career should be based on his patients' stories. Chapter 2 provides descriptions of some patients from his clinical records. These case histories are presented uncut as Freeman wrote them for a general audience.

It should be stressed that, when one is dealing with traumatic brain injury, no two patients are identical. In this respect, such injuries differ from many medical conditions in which it is possible, on the basis of clinical observation and laboratory investigation, to gain a comprehensive understanding of the nature of the pathological changes underlying those conditions. The likelihood of heterogeneity in pathology among patients who present similar clinical features of brain injury may impede such understanding. Limitations in understanding the natural history of repair in the injured brain presented another obstacle to any attempts to undertake scientifically plausible and interpretable clinical trials of Freeman's practices. Any clinical trial, if its results are to be subject to interpretation, requires that like is being compared with like.

The clinical histories to be recounted each illustrate a number of features of the experiences of patients with brain injury. The selection of the term 'experience' in relation to these patients is quite deliberate, notwithstanding a commonly expressed opinion that they are, *by definition*, incapable of experience. Reading of some patient histories, I suggest, cannot fail to raise doubts about the value of 'commonly expressed opinion'. None of the patients whose stories are to be recounted will exemplify exclusively the point that she or he has been selected to illustrate. After reading two dozen histories, I have selected a group because their stories provide a good account of particular aspects.

The points chosen for presentation and emphasis include the frequent inadequacy of clinical assessment of the patient's level of awareness and the resultant precipitate consignment of affected individuals to aged-care facilities. A consequence of these events has been the aggravation of co-morbidities that are likely to confound any belated attempts at neurological rehabilitation. Attention will also be directed in the case histories to the essential requirement of a highly motivated family when embarking on rehabilitation and to provide examples of the manner in which family commitment can enable rehabilitation of a disabled member.

Freeman learnt much, not only from his patients, but also from their families. The most cursory reading of his case histories will reveal the extent to which unstinting commitment of immediate family members, accompanied frequently by scores of volunteers, to home-based rehabilitation programs designed and overseen by Freeman was critical. On one occasion in the mid 1990s, a large group of people who had participated in such programs wrote individual letters recounting their experiences. Chapter 3 contains extracts from some of these letters. They have been composed by people with a broad range of educational and socioeconomic backgrounds, but they display, in common, a 'hands-on' comprehension of the realities of living with acquired brain injury over many years. Notwithstanding this ongoing burden, they contain many examples of the triumph of the human spirit.

The carers' stories, being a thoroughly realistic lay account of brain injury, include many details of non-medical aspects such as financial perils, litigation over accidents and intra-familial stress. Whilst these accoutrements merit wide exposure in the community, the present account will generally be restricted to extracts dealing with more clinical aspects.

Chapters 4 and 5 deal with two discrete issues that require a separation that they frequently have not been accorded. The loosely applied expression 'coma arousal' misleadingly lumps the detection of an individual's retained or regained level of awareness after a brain injury together with the outcomes of subsequent efforts at rehabilitation that aim, among other goals, to enhance that awareness. To emphasise the importance I attach to drawing the distinction between the implications of the first return of consciousness (or, more accurately, its ascertainment by others) and subsequent stages of recovery, the two issues are dealt with in separate chapters.

The inevitable connection between the two topics is that the attitudes of others towards the individual, and the course of management to be adopted, will be strongly influenced by the prevailing impression about the patient's level of awareness. There are abundant and uncontested reports in the medical literature of the considerable incidence of incorrect diagnosis of vegetative states. The adjective 'vegetative' had already been conferred by other medical practitioners on many of the people coming under Freeman's care. His experience—much of it reported in peer-reviewed, overseas medical journals—was that both the nature and the usual circumstances of a conventional neurological examination were inappropriate to detect or exclude awareness. The strategy of the clinical examination that he developed to detect any signs of awareness is presented in Chapter 4. With the benefit of a quarter-century of research, especially that based on technologically refined brain scanning, it is possible to gain an insight into the scientific basis of some of Freeman's observations.

Chapter 5 will consider the evolution of the approach that Ted Freeman developed to facilitate the further rehabilitation of people who, after emerging from coma, remained severely limited. This evolution, underpinned by his conviction that hope remained after severe brain injury, even when this is followed by prolonged unconsciousness, impacted upon the Australian medical scene. Essentially, this entailed the interaction of a man and his ideas with an established system based on different beliefs.

In most instances, a medical practitioner espousing a philosophy and resultant clinical approach that is at variance with traditionally embedded practice (unless she or he had already attained a leadership position in the profession—clinical, academic or administrative) could find it difficult to apply beyond a personal medical practice. Several factors contributed to producing an exception in the case of Freeman: of these, the most influential undoubtedly was money.

The commonest cause of acquired brain injury among younger people remains motor vehicle accidents. Frequently, these generate large insurance claims, which, in the case of young individuals, may entail many decades of expensive high-care support. Any variation in management that offered the possibility of lower levels of support for lesser periods clearly has the potential to reduce compensation costs. In fairness to insurance industry people who made the decision to fund the implementation of Freeman's ideas, it is likely that simple humanitarian precepts were also influential.

A second source of impetus for the introduction of his ideas into medical systems were the people who feature in Chapter 3—namely, families and friends of patients. By the nature of living with a family member afflicted with brain injury, this group had limited time to agitate for change. Finally, from his account of events, it is clear that some medical, nursing and paramedical personnel were appalled at the warehousing of patients with brain injury and sought any viable alternative.

An issue that ran alongside Freeman's work for two decades was that of conducting a trial to prove or disprove his claims. This history, which is central to any understanding of his experiences, is outlined in Chapter 6. Fundamental to the concept of evidence-based medicine is a requirement to establish the efficacy and safety of any proposed novel treatment irrespective of whether it is based on drugs, surgical intervention, physical therapy or whatever. Efficacy requires a demonstration of its superiority over the currently best available alternative measures.

The preferred strategy to establish superiority of novel therapies is to conduct a randomised control trial. Two attributes of such trials, insofar as they relate to recovery from coma, are examined—namely, their efficacy and their ethical soundness. The chequered history of proposals to mount such a trial of Freeman's practices is also reviewed. Whilst Freeman attracted opposition from some of his neurosurgical and rehabilitation colleagues for his views, he increasingly came to be at the mercy of some other, more academically positioned, colleagues who specialised in conducting clinical trials. To express it bluntly, such colleagues were often eager to obtain the funding that Freeman and his patients' families had secured but preferred not to involve him in the research to which it was to be applied.

Chapter 7 will examine the basis for, and the nature of, the opposition that Freeman encountered. The simplest interpretation for this opposition would appear to be that Freeman was treading on the patch of a number of medical specialties in which he lacked the requisite formal qualifications. He was also, by implication, condemning the systemic approach to patients deemed to be irreversibly unconscious. There existed, and still largely exists, a hiatus in medical responsibility for these people. To a considerable extent, this may reflect the dominance of a curative medical model that disdains evidence considered to be 'non-scientific'.

Australian neurosurgeons, and intensivists in their turn, generally maintain a standard comparable with the best in the world but, once the initial period after brain injury has passed, they are out of the game. A disconnect can arise between high-intensity procedures with curative goals and rehabilitative care. Rehabilitation services are of variable quality but, with few exceptions, their entry requirements for treatment cannot be met by many brain injured patients—a strategy colloquially referred to as picking winners. As to the form taken by opposition to Ted Freeman, this ranged from the decidedly petty to the most damaging form—namely, vigorous defamation under parliamentary privilege.

Chapter 8 presents another set of assessments of Freeman's work. In contrast with the preceding chapter, which recounts some of the Australian reactions against him, this chapter is largely concerned with international appraisal of his achievements. This contrasts again with Chapter 7 in that, overwhelmingly, these were very positive. Interestingly, the assessments of overseas clinicians were as instrumental in accomplishing the reversal of the parliamentary defamation referred to above as Australian assessments, frequently anonymous, had been in fuelling that defamation.

Chapter 9, a short postscript, reflects briefly on several factors that impacted on the evolution of Freeman's approach to rehabilitation after brain injury, especially the entrenched attitudes of some colleagues and their reticence to countenance alternative responses to this problem. The discussion will look forward towards opportunities to remedy the systemic failures of the medical system that were experienced by many families. These opportunities centre on the proposed Australian National Disability Insurance Scheme (NDIS). If the NDIS is successfully implemented, major beneficiaries are likely to be future patients and their families who are confronted with the situations that characterised Freeman's families.

1. The origins of a commitment

In order to place Ted Freeman's career path in context, I asked him to describe his background leading up to his first involvement with people with brain injuries. This chapter is his response. He prefaced that description with a quotation:

> What we are today comes from our thoughts of yesterday.
> And our present thoughts build our life of tomorrow.
>
> — The Buddha

He told the following story.

In 1949 at the age of sixteen I worked pushing a barrow at the Sydney City Markets. I had been a schoolboy at Canterbury Boy's High School in Sydney—a selective high school whose motto is 'Truth and Honour'. In the 1950s, few students went to university. Most school-leavers worked in the public service, the police force or the commercial world of shops, offices, banks and insurance companies—the so-called white-collar jobs. Others went into trades as blue-collar workers or became labourers like me. As a schoolboy, I can recall riding in a tram past the imposing sandstone gates of the University of Sydney, looking at the students and thinking I would never be able to enter a university. I wondered how people without money could ever study there. My family had none.

My father, an Englishman, came to Australia in October 1911. He joined the 18th Battalion, 5th Brigade, 2nd Division of the AIF and was wounded by shrapnel at Gallipoli in 1915 at the notorious 'Hill 60' when, as raw recruits, they were given orders to assault an entrenched Turkish position with bayonets. He later fought at Bullecourt on the Somme in 1916 and at Passchendaele in the Third Battle of Ypres in 1917 where he sustained a gunshot wound to his right leg. An above-knee amputation was later performed. In the days before modern anaesthetics, blood transfusions, antibiotics and resuscitation, the mortality from such a wound and operation was high, often 25 per cent. My parents met in Sydney when my father was in Rose Hall, a Red Cross rehabilitation facility.

My mother was a country girl from the far northern NSW town of Mullumbimby where her father, Charles Alfred Shepherd, was the veterinary surgeon. He had served in the Veterinary Corps in the Boer War and my mother had been named 'Victoria Mafeking'. She was invariably known as 'Maffie' to family and friends. Country girls came to Rose Hall to help with the general care of the returned soldiers. My parents were married in 1929. Some sedentary occupations were specifically reserved for disabled soldiers and my father became a lift attendant at an insurance company in Sydney. We lived in a War Service Home. My father died in 1937 leaving my mother to raise my brothers Bill, aged seven, and John and I (twins), aged four.

When our father was dying, John and I were placed for six months in Burnside Presbyterian Homes, an orphanage at Parramatta. Neither John nor I can recall a great deal of this time at Burnside but when I look at my grandchildren I wonder how such fragile and tender young children do survive what for us was in effect the loss of both father and mother during that time. My mother had to return to work to support the family. In those days women were paid roughly half the male wage so it was a constant struggle for her. But she was a courageous woman who loved us with a passion and maintained her good humour through all her difficulties.

One day my mother questioned me about my future. 'Have you thought about what you are going to do with your life? Have you thought about going to university?' She suggested that I apply to the Sydney Technical College to study for the Leaving Certificate. I enjoyed the learning process and did well enough to gain a Commonwealth University Scholarship. This provided for my university fees and a small living allowance while studying at the medical school at the University of Sydney. Early in my studies I met a gorgeous girl, Dorothy Thomson. She and I were married in 1956. It has remained a love match as we have journeyed through life together. It was unusual for a student to be married. Some distant members of my family reminded me of cousin 'so and so' who had failed at university when he married. But we were both happy and I passed all the exams.

Money was short. We did have a job cleaning the local church and Dorothy played the organ for weddings and funerals as well as teaching some music students. If things became really difficult I would work as a brickie's labourer or at whatever job I could find during university recess.

After graduation in January 1959, I gained a broad experience of most facets of medicine by working for four years in hospitals in New South Wales, Queensland and Papua and New Guinea. At the end of 1963 I took the position as Medical Superintendent of the Paton Memorial Hospital, a Presbyterian Mission hospital in Port Vila, the capital of the New Hebrides, now Vanuatu. The New Hebrides at that time was an undeveloped group of islands in the South-West Pacific jointly controlled by Britain and France. This form of government was known as the Condominium, although ironically called the 'Pandemonium' by the locals and expatriates.[1]

---

1 Marney Dunn (1997) *Pandemonium or Paradise*. Crawford House, Bathurst, NSW.

My time in Port Vila exposed me to a wide range of medical, surgical, obstetric and paediatric problems and some diseases not seen by medical practitioners in developed countries. Malaria, pneumonia, tuberculosis, dysentery and meningitis were rife. Leprosy also occurred on some of the islands. The hospital had excellent Australian and New Zealand mission nursing sisters but inadequate funds and often depended on donations from voluntary organisations like the Red Cross for equipment and pharmaceutical drugs to continue to provide a service to the people of the New Hebrides, both indigenous and expatriate.[2]

Microscopic pathology was limited to slides for tuberculosis, malaria parasites, spinal taps and anaemia. X-rays were used to examine fractured limbs and for the detection of pneumonia or tuberculosis in the lungs. Much of the success of my medical work depended on close visual observation of the patient and using my hands to feel, palpate and percuss in order to make a clinical diagnosis. These classical methods of inspection, palpation, percussion and auscultation, which have been taught to medical students throughout centuries, have now been superseded by laboratory investigations, sometimes to the disadvantage of the patient. Young physicians seem confused about physical examination. Together with the (clinical) history, physical examination is the doctor's best-kept secret: powerful, portable, fast, cheap, durable, reproducible and fun.

While I was at Paton Memorial Hospital the British Administration sought and obtained a grant from the World Health Organisation (WHO) for me to study surgery in Edinburgh—the oldest surgical school in the world and one with a first-rate reputation. The British intended to build a new hospital in Port Vila and offered me the post of medical superintendent. Dorothy and I packed up the family of six children and went to Scotland in December 1968. I studied hard and completed the Fellowship of the Royal College of Surgeons of Edinburgh (FRCSE) and returned to Vanuatu early in 1970.

Some months after my return I was performing a caesarean on a patient with an obstructed labour. I began to sweat profusely and, with a severe headache and tremors, I thought I had malaria, although I had taken my preventative drug, Chloroquine. I developed a stiff neck and I began to fear meningitis, which was confirmed by lumbar puncture performed by the excellent New Hebridean doctor Dr Makau Kalsakau.

I can vaguely recall early one morning being taken by stretcher on a small boat from the hospital on Iririki to the Vila Airport where the Royal Australian Air Force had a Hercules air transport waiting. Noise protectors were placed on my ears, and I was given an injection. I have no recollection of the trip or arrival at Sydney Airport.

---

2   Edward Freeman (2001) *Doctor in Vanuatu*. University of the South Pacific, Suva.

I awoke in Sydney Hospital in a back room adjacent to the intensive therapy unit, since the doctors thought I might be infectious. The room was obviously the storage area for the unit and I was alone. Night closed in. I was too weak to eat the food. It was May, the weather was cold and I had come straight from the tropics. I lost body heat and began to shiver and desperately wanted more blankets. A bell had been placed on a bedside table, but it was out of my reach. I yelled as loudly as I could for help, but no-one heard.

Hours later a nurse came into the storeroom, looked at me in surprise and said, 'What are you doing here?' I had been forgotten. She gave me some warm blankets. The weakness I experienced is difficult to describe. It was past fatigue. Just as a person can be mentally desolate, I am sure that the body can be physically desolate. I had no power. The effort of breathing seemed to take all my strength. Any other action was superfluous. To move an arm or a leg or to attempt to sit up or to eat took enormous concentration and effort and resulted in extreme fatigue. The only people I wanted to see were my wife and immediate family.

After some weeks, I had finished my antibiotics, my lumbar puncture results were improving and no further treatment was necessary. Over the days, I urged my wife to 'get me out'. I couldn't wait to get home even though it was only to a small mission flat in an inner western Sydney suburb.

I learnt two things from my illness. First, the experience wrote into my brain what it would be like to be disabled, to be so locked into one's body like Annie, who wrote that being in an institution 'removes all hope'.[3] Second, I realised that the best place for the sick person, if at all possible, is home.

A year later I was appointed the Medical Superintendent of the Gosford District Hospital on the Central Coast of New South Wales. Gosford was a burgeoning town close enough to Sydney to be a commuter suburb. The position was mainly medical administration with a small clinical component. Excellent doctors served the patients in the hospital. This was in the time of the honorary medical system when the doctors proudly gave their time unstintingly to both public and private patients. I remained in this position for five years before going into general practice.

One day in 1979 a mother came into my consulting room. Her five-year-old daughter had an ear infection. The little girl had suffered cerebral palsy from birth and could not talk. Medical schools did not teach about the conditions of cerebral palsy or Down syndrome. These two conditions tended to be lumped together as an unfortunate fact of life and the children were regarded as being

---

3   Anne Macdonald & Rose Crossley (1980) *Annie's Coming Out*. Penguin, Melbourne.

mentally defective and were often placed in mental institutions or hospitals for the developmentally delayed. The medical opinion was that nothing could be done for them.

But this child seemed to communicate with her mother. With increasing curiosity, I questioned myself, 'What is going on here? This is an unusual scene. Is this mother really getting through to her child? Am I missing something and, if so, what? Can I learn something here?' I left the surgery that evening puzzled over what I had seen. I described the consultation to Dorothy when I arrived home. She said to me, 'You are obviously intrigued. What are you going to do about it?' I replied, 'I don't know.' Shortly after this episode I met the grandfather of a child with cerebral palsy. He was raising funds to send his grandchild to the United States for treatment at the Institutes for the Achievement of Human Potential (IAHP) in Philadelphia. I inquired about this institution. My medical and educational colleagues warned me strongly against the institutes, which were not recognised by the medical profession. They told me the institutes had produced no scientific evidence to back up the claim they could help children with brain injury. They said the institutes provided false hope and treatment was expensive. While the word charlatan was not used, this was the message. I was advised not to go. But I was interested. I wrote to the institutes and asked if I might visit. The reply was welcoming.

Dorothy and I left Sydney in June 1979, landed in Vancouver and bussed overland to Philadelphia. Since I was experienced in clinical and administrative work in both developed and undeveloped countries, I thought I only needed a short time there, perhaps a day or two. Dr Glenn Doman, the founder of the institutes and the author of a well-known book on brain injury in children, was originally a physical therapist and had worked previously in partnership with an educationist, Dr Delacato, but the two had separated.[4] Dr Doman greeted me warmly. When I asked him about the question of outcomes, he answered, 'You can have access to all our files and do as much research as you like to see our results.' I did not think this would be any help since I knew very little about brain injury—a subject never taught at medical school.

I was shown around the centre and finally introduced to a very senior physician, Dr Edward Le Winn, MD, FACP, formerly the senior attending physician emeritus (chief) of the Albert Einstein Medical Centre in Philadelphia. Dr Le Winn's honest and positive but careful attitude to the children with brain injury intrigued me. I left the institutes late in the afternoon and when I arrived back at the hotel I said to Dorothy, 'I would like to revise our plans and stay in Philadelphia longer.' I went for the next four days to the institutes. The repeated

---

4   Glenn Doman (1974) *What to Do about Your Brain Injured Child*. Doubleday, New York.

message was that much could be done to help the person with a brain injury but it required time and effort and resources. Without these inputs there could be no improvement.

Each day I met with Le Winn and examined children, discussing with him their initial problems, their potential and possibilities for improvement. I watched as therapy was tailored specifically for each child. The dedication of the families impressed me and also their grasp on the realities of their problems. I did not see any evidence that these parents were given false hope. Rather, they were encouraged to look at what may be possible. At this interval, I am reminded of the conclusion to a 1995 article: 'It is not too many years ago that students were taught that the human nerve cell is so highly specialised that it cannot repair itself.'[5] Our teachers were wrong.

The central philosophy of the institutes was that the dynamic potential—that is, spare capacity—of the injured brain to improve is enormous and it is important to redevelop certain areas of the brain in order to obtain improvement. The brain has to be worked in the same way that a muscle needs to be worked. If the brain is not worked it will atrophy (shrink).

This change in the brain cells has now been termed 'plasticity'. In those days the term was either not invented or rarely used. Its significance for those with a brain injury is immense because the injured brain does not suddenly become rock-hard and solid. There is no reason to suppose that the injured brain loses the ability to change and regain some function if it is given the correct environment. In other words, the injured brain can be reorganised by providing the optimum environment. Neurological reorganisation was the basis of the institutes' work.

The other concept that the institutes promoted is that the correct way to regain function is by redeveloping the most primitive areas of the brain and building a pattern of development on this basis. Just as the developing infant learns to push back in the bassinet, then roll over onto his/her front, then push along the floor on his/her abdomen, then lift his/her head from the floor and rise up onto hands and knees, then crawl, then stand holding onto a support structure, then cruise from one piece of furniture to the next and then walk with the arms held out to balance before walking freely without support, so, the person with a brain injury may need to go through the same stages as they recover. This developmental approach has many other supporters. It fits in with the work of Piaget, Gesell and other well-known developmentalists. It is rather like building a house by laying the foundations first before the superstructure is placed in position.

---

5   Donald G. Stein, Simon Brailowsky & Bruno Will (1995) *Brain Repair*. Oxford University Press, Oxford.

I found much to be genuine at the institutes both in the people and in their methods. I could not discount the work I had witnessed there. It whetted my appetite to explore further. Much of what I discovered later as an independent researcher supported the work of the institutes.

Dorothy and I returned to Australia from Philadelphia. The medical group practice where I worked was large and demanding and the questions raised in my mind in Philadelphia about brain injury were soon swamped by more pressing demands on my time.

But on Thursday, 10 April 1980 our lives changed totally and forever. While I was playing tennis with some friends a police car arrived and told us that our eldest son, Matthew, had been killed in a road accident. We both started crying in disbelief. Ross, our youngest son, was also present. We gathered him up and drove home totally overwhelmed with grief and loss. You never think that such a thing is going to happen to a member of your family. Our children as well as Dorothy and I were heartbroken.

We made arrangements for Matthew's funeral. We intended to see his body but the undertaker rang to say that it would be better not to. He had sustained a severe head injury and was killed instantly. The editor of the local newspaper, whom I knew well, rang up for information about the accident. He asked, 'How is Dorothy?' I said, 'All right.' What else can you say? Talk seemed pointless. He then said to me, 'You will be all right, Ted, since you are used to this sort of thing'! He meant death of course. I was amazed, for he was a kindly man.

I did not go to work for a week. Dorothy and I went to the beach each day and sat. There was not much conversation between us. What could we talk about that was of any significance beside the catastrophe that had struck our family? On about the fifth day after Matt's death I said to Dorothy, 'I feel that there is something special for me to do.' Almost instantly, I knew that I had to research brain injury.

I am a firm believer in the concept of the 'wounded healer'. I believe it is possible that the person who is wounded can turn that hurt from a negative to a positive. The strength that arises from experience of this pain can be used to minister to other people passing through a similar episode. I am not a pastor, priest or minister and my strength does not lie in that direction but I had been and could be a healer. That much I knew. On the back cover of Father Henri Nouwen's book are the words:

> It is his [Nouwen's] contention that the minister is called to recognise the sufferings of his time in his own heart and make that recognition

the starting point of his service. In other words, the minister must be willing to go beyond his professional role and leave himself open as a fellow human being with the same wounds and sufferings.[6]

I knew I must learn more about brain injury and find my professional role in helping both the patients and their families. I approached a friend in the Department of Health, Dr Ted Cullen. I told him I wanted to work with patients who had been brain injured. He was supportive but explained there was not much work or research being done with patients diagnosed as brain injured. He did say, 'This is probably not what you want but there is a position at Peat Island Hospital.'

Peat Island was a hospital on the Hawkesbury River for people with mental retardation and developmental delay. I regarded it as being at the lowest point in medicine, but a friend said, 'Ted, you haven't tried it yet. How do you know if you don't try?'

In January 1981, I met with the Medical Superintendent of Peat Island and walked around the wards with him. There were approximately 160 patients, or residents as they were called. Some had been inmates for almost 50 years. The staff were caring but it was a custodial institution. Many of the wards had an open-door policy. One ward did not. It was Ward Four. Its doors were heavily padlocked and the windows had heavy wire mesh over them. It was a prison. The smell of human urine, faeces and vomit hit you the moment you entered. The patients were shouting, screaming, yelling, banging their heads, jostling each other, walking or dragging themselves from one place to another apparently without purpose. Many had adopted the typical institutional constant rocking movement—backwards and forwards—whether standing, sitting or lying on the seats or on the floor. Some were openly aggressive. It was *One Flew over the Cuckoo's Nest* in reality.

Most of the nurses, male and female, genuinely cared for the people. At no stage did I see any staff member physically abuse any resident. It was the healthcare system that was at fault. The staff were caught in the system to the same extent as the residents except they had those two irreplaceable advantages—power and freedom—both denied to the inmates. I took a deep breath of fresh air each day as I walked away from Ward Four to rid the smell from my nostrils and the noise and sights from my brain. I realised that if I was put in Ward Four as a resident I would go mad. The environment would destroy me as I am sure it did those unfortunate people.

I researched the medical records of each patient in Ward Four. One-third of admissions were post encephalitis, often from measles; one-third were admitted

6   Henri Nouwen (1979) *The Wounded Healer.* Image Books, New York.

because of cerebral palsy. No information was recorded about the other inmates. I noted many records on incidental things such as skin rash or ingrowing toenails or haemorrhoids but only minor entries detailing the brain injury or the mental state or behaviour of the inmates. The data were very unbalanced. The clinical notes indicated no therapy had been given even on a trial basis in Ward Four. The residents in this ward were there forever. For them, death was the only release. There were diversionary programs for residents in other wards of the hospital. The actual objectives of the programs were difficult to determine. Mostly, it seemed they were 'revolving-door' programs, which meant the residents did the program and finished in precisely the same position as they were in when they started.

In its fully functioning period a decade or so before, Peat Island and an adjoining island, Milson Island, had a total of 650 residents. Three doctors would certainly have been needed but the establishment for medical officers had not been reduced with the decreased patient load. The island was heavily over-doctored. The Medical Superintendent was a very kind man near retirement age. He attended the hospital every weekday and ran a general practice clinic for minor ailments. There was another doctor, who had an inquiring mind and who gave me considerable help. And then there was me—three doctors for 160 patients, most of whom were not physically sick.

I soon realised that there was little work for me to do. A small office in the front room of the former mortuary became available for me. I started a program of learning and research. Every morning I arrived at 8.30 and after checking on some of the wards I moved into my room and studied my books and journals for hours each day. Where to begin was the difficulty. My only information was from the institutes in Philadelphia. Just to mention their name produced a highly emotional, antagonistic and at times aggressive reaction in both medical and educational circles. Also, the National Health and Medical Research Council (NHMRC) in Australia had issued a report that stated that there was no scientific basis for the work of the institutes (this, of course, was true in 1976).[7]

I decided to research normal brain function and after that consider the effects of a brain injury. I read every piece of literature I could find relating to brain function and brain injury. By the end of 1981 three concepts appeared to provide a theoretical and possibly practical approach to helping people with brain injury. They were canalisation—that is, the inherent pathway of development and redevelopment of the brain—the enormous spare capacity of the brain, and the neuroplasticity of the brain.

---

7 National Health and Medical Research Council (1976) *Report of the Therapeutic Goods Subcommittee to Investigate the Methods used by the Institutes for the Achievement of Human potential*. 82nd Session of Council.

While I was working at Peat Island I met Ian Hunter, the Clinical Director of the Australian Centre for Brain Injured Children (ACBIC). Ian came from Melbourne, where his centre was located, but he travelled around the capital cities of Australia and consulted with families whose children had suffered a brain injury. Ian had trained in Philadelphia at the Institutes for the Achievement of Human Potential. Whenever Ian came to Sydney we discussed programs and therapies. I found him to be responsible, conscientious and honest in all his dealings with the patients and their relatives and I learnt much from him as I sat in on his clinics and watched his approach.

It was Socrates who first said that questions are more important than answers. Only questions, he said, could keep people intellectually honest.

Transferring answers from one brain to another has fairly predictable consequences: answers are safe. Infecting minds with questions is hazardous: it is impossible to predict the outcome.

I was preparing a paper on coma when *The Lancet* published a letter by Dr Le Winn and Dr Mihai Dimancescu, a New York neurosurgeon who had established a coma recovery unit in the United States.[8] They gave quite startling and positive results from a small group of comatose patients they had treated using increased environmental stimulation. Le Winn sent me a copy of his paper, which detailed his method of sensory stimulation in the patient in coma.

At this time the attitude of the administration at Peat Island changed. The Area General Medical Superintendent called me into his office one afternoon. He appeared to be very annoyed. He asked, 'Did you know that your name had been linked with Ian Hunter and his organisation [ACBIC]?' I said, 'Yes, that is possible.' He told me it was against Health Commission policy to be associated with this organisation. He demanded to know what scientific proof they possessed. I listened to him quietly and then said, 'Come with me and I will show you what your so-called scientific principles have produced. I will open the door of Ward Four and you can look inside. That is what your scientific principles have done.' He finally said, 'I forbid you to have anything more to do with Ian Hunter. You are not to see him again.' I said, 'I'm sorry. I cannot agree with your request', and I left his office.

I was not the only one asking questions. There were other people seeking to expose the failure of the health system to fulfil its duty of care to similar patients. Peter McLean, the previous secretary of the NSW Subnormal Children's Welfare Association, produced a report on Stockton Hospital, an institution with 830 residents. He wrote: 'I am still finding it difficult to cope with what I can only

---

8   Edward Le Winn & Mihai Dimanescu (1978) Sensory enrichment in coma. *The Lancet, ii*, 156.

call an appalling state of affairs at Stockton Hospital.'[9] He writes of the lack of staff, that the children sense their 'aloneness and rejection', that some children were 'self mutilating', and that 'some children never left their wards'. McLean finished:

> I have not written about the abuse and deprivation of just one child in an isolated case. I am writing about 300 children in just one place alone. How many other institutions in this state are doing more or less the same thing to handicapped children. It may be better to replace the word 'state' with the all-embracing word 'country'.

I asked a variety of people to come to Peat Island to observe the condition of the patients. They were psychologists, physicians, ministers of religion and politicians. All were appalled, but there seemed to be no authority that could actually expose the conditions and resolve some of the problems.

I desperately needed a group of reputable people to whom I could report. At the suggestion of a friend, a support group was formed to keep me 'in balance' and, as much as possible, out of trouble. One friend who agreed to join the group warned me that 'you are in a difficult work area. The road ahead will be hard.' Dr Malcolm Mackay, a former minister in the Menzies Government, became the chairman. Malcolm had a deep and personal commitment to the research as his own daughter Elsbeth had died following a traumatic brain injury. Two Sydney businessmen, a former moderator-general of the Presbyterian Church of Australia and a physician colleague completed the group.

There was general agreement among the members that the letter published in *The Lancet* on the subject of coma by Le Winn and Dimancescu might be the way forward. The committee reasoned that traumatic brain injury was different from brain injury in childbirth. Traumatic brain injury involved a situation where a once healthy and vibrant person with full faculties was suddenly altered by one accident. Unlike the situation with brain injury present since birth, lifestyle and abilities had already been established.

Following my confrontation with the Area General Medical Superintendent, I realised that I was in serious difficulty at Peat Island. I still had research to do. I did not want to leave, but I knew the axe must fall. I had challenged the healthcare system. I had questioned the authorities who controlled my employment. I was regarded as a troublesome heretic. The pay scales for doctors on my grade at Peat Island were very low and the financial upkeep of our five children was considerable. We were not lavish spenders, rather the reverse. Our lifestyle was simple. I spoke to Dorothy about the importance of the work on brain injury. She knew a great deal about it since I constantly discussed

---

9   Peter McLean (1981) *Report on Stockton Hospital*. NSW Subnormal Children's Association, Sydney.

with her the events of each day. She expressed concern, however, that I was so immersed in the study of severe brain injury that it was dominating our lives. But I continued to do the research. I finished a paper on coma incorporating the new knowledge I had acquired and sent it to a selection of medical people. Some thought my document could be worthwhile, but more research needed to be done.

An arrangement was made for me to meet with a neurologist and a rehabilitation specialist. The neurologist had an open mind and positive approach, but he also quite reasonably suggested that further investigation and research were needed. The rehabilitation specialist was not receptive. When I met him in his office he had not bothered to read the paper. I soon found that he had a very narrow concept of what could be done with people who have been brain injured. He told me: 'No matter what you do for them, they just keep coming back. They are part of the "revolving door" syndrome.' He said, 'You should be working out how to retire rather than delve into areas about which you are totally ignorant.' I was kept on at Peat Island as long as possible, but finally that position was terminated.

In March 1982 I went to Melbourne to observe Ian Hunter at work and to learn more from him. Once again I had a demonstration of how difficult it is for the medical profession to deal with alternative thinking. I invited a medical friend to come to the ACBIC clinic. He arrived late and was obviously distressed. He told me that his colleagues in his medical practice objected strongly to his coming to an organisation that was not accepted by orthodox medicine. He had argued with them and finally walked away from them in disgust at their attitude.

On returning to Sydney, I approached various organisations for support. I prepared a copy of my paper on the new approach to coma and submitted it to the NSW Government Insurance Office (GIO). The Chief Medical Officer expressed interest in the document. GIO paid large sums of insurance money to those people who had survived severe brain injury. It made sense to reduce the extent of injury if possible and therefore lessen the payout amounts.

I spoke to many Rotary clubs about the problems of the children who were in places like Peat Island. Each time I finished my address, concerned Rotarians came to talk with me in order to find out what they could do. Sometimes awkward situations occurred. My speech was still very much based on the findings of my work at Peat Island and the disregard that the government and medical profession showed towards these unfortunate children. I always quoted part of the report from December 1981 by McLean of the Subnormal Children's Welfare Association and also the comments from the report of the Anti-Discrimination Board of New South Wales:

The failure of public policy has been to render people with intellectual handicaps virtually second-class citizens and arguably the most impoverished and underprivileged group in our society. If the test of a society is how it treats its poorest, most marginal people, then the findings in the report indicate that our society is seriously wanting.[10]

After I had given the speech a few dozen times, I knew it by heart and rarely referred to my notes. Before one of the biggest and most powerful Rotary clubs in the country, when my eye roamed around the audience, I caught sight of a collection of medical administrators responsible for the hospital and health service that I was attacking. One administrator had been delegated to give the vote of thanks. He was very sparse in his comments and our meeting afterwards was frosty; however, there was a great deal of goodwill from the Rotary clubs in general. They all expressed interest and wanted to help, but no-one seemed to know what to do.

Malcolm Mackay, the chair of my support group, had been appointed as a consultant to World Vision, the large and very effective international charity that supports people in underdeveloped countries. Malcolm arranged a meeting in Melbourne with the Executive Director of World Vision. He sought the opinion of a medical consultant, which was very positive. Some days later, early in June 1982, Malcolm Mackay invited me to another meeting with World Vision. The organisation had decided that my work could benefit those with brain injury in underdeveloped countries as well as in Australia and therefore would support me. The support, which would begin immediately, would not be a professional wage but more of a stipend, paid six monthly, as well as a small expense account to provide for travel and accommodation costs; but it was enough to keep my family afloat.

I usually get to sleep easily and sleep very well. That night in Melbourne, I was so excited I lay in bed with myriad thoughts churning through my mind. I suppose the uppermost thoughts were thankfulness and gratitude and I couldn't wait to get home to tell Dorothy. Now I could continue with the work. The Executive Director of World Vision gave me a letter of introduction:

World Vision has taken up the challenge to enlist support for Dr Freeman so that he can continue his investigation into the most recent developments in the field of brain injury to children.

In the course of our worldwide care for children suffering from the effects of poverty, malnutrition, war and violence, we are continually confronted with multitudes of children suffering from what many feel to

---

10 NSW Anti-Discrimination Board (1981) *Discrimination of the Intellectually Handicapped*. NSW Anti-Discrimination Board, Sydney.

be irreparable brain damage. This moves us to seek for any possibility of treatment which might enable these children to be released from a living prison and take up useful and meaningful lives.

A Health Commission official offered some office accommodation and also research facilities in his building. He did make some reasonable requests: that traditional scientific procedures should be followed and that the name of the commission could only be used with their specific authority and no publications should be issued without their approval. It looked like I was on the way at last. Funding and some semblance of credibility, even though small, had arrived.

I now began working in earnest on the research into coma. Two generations ago a coma that lasted for more than a couple of days would have been virtually unknown because the patient would have died. It is my belief that nowadays, because modern medicine keeps people alive by artificial means, patients can survive in coma for weeks and months. Medical technology has provided the ventilator, which can breathe for them, fluid is provided through intravenous lines and urine is drained away by catheter. Tubes inserted through the abdominal wall directly into the stomach (gastrostomy tubes) provide food.

I soon found that there was a considerable body of medical opinion that regarded coma as a sleep-like protective state and that nothing should be done to the person in coma, apart from general nursing care. The patient should be placed in a darkened room and allowed to sleep, during which time the brain would heal itself. Many orthodox doctors supported this theory and would not listen to opinions to the contrary.

At one medical meeting I spoke to the keynote speaker, a professor, about the possibility that this passive approach should be challenged, as it was well documented that the longer a patient remained in coma the worse was their outcome.[11] I suggested to him that coma victims were being placed in extreme sensory deprivation by three factors: their injuries, the poor sensory input from their environment and the heavy use of sedative drugs. His face went very red. He said, 'You are totally wrong', and turned away. He refused further discussion. I found this attitude to be quite common.

A marker event now took place. The Regional Director from the Northern Region of the Health Commission referred me to the Royal North Shore Hospital in Sydney with a request to allow me to have access to the medical records of those patients who had suffered brain injury during the preceding three years for a new approach to the patient in coma. I was introduced to two specialists there. One was an epidemiologist—that is, a person who is skilled in plotting the

---

11   Carl Carlsson, Claes von Essen & Jan Lofgren (1968) Factors affecting the clinical outcome of patients with severe head injury. *Neurosurgery, 129*, 242.

results of changing factors in a statistical group of people or a community and who can structure research projects correctly. The epidemiologist, being non-medical, had an open mind on the subject. The other was a psychiatrist who had done pioneering work observing changes in the immune system caused by the body's reaction to grief.

Both were interested in the research. They considered it a legitimate field of study. It made sense to these two doctors that the patient should be given a structured input of stimulation to achieve arousal rather than leaving the patient to lie in bed in a state of sensory deprivation with no or minimal therapy. The question was how could this reawakening of the brain be undertaken? There were several alternatives but the most natural process was to provide an input to the brain through the senses of vision, hearing, touch, smell and movement.

In late 1982, I was asked to contact Kevin Beckton, the Assistant General Manager (Legal) at GIO, for an appointment. I saw Kevin soon after. When the niceties of introduction were finished, Kevin asked, 'What do you want?' Kevin is one of those no-nonsense people, disarming and very shrewd. He had spent many years involved in investigating claims made to the GIO by people who had suffered accidents and he had helped to establish a spinal unit in Sydney. We discussed the research. I explained that my funding was from World Vision. I said that World Vision would be delighted if GIO relieved them of the funding requirement.

The General Manager of GIO indicated that they were interested in offering a contract. I accepted an offer. Dorothy and I later repaid World Vision all of the money we had received from them. The research gained support at the board meeting of the GIO and things were really on a roll. The NSW GIO had size, status, authority and money. A letter on GIO letterhead gave immediate and substantial credence to the research:

GOVERNMENT INSURANCE OFFICE OF N.S.W.
153–163 PHILLIP STREET, Sydney

Dear Sir,

Dr. E. Freeman MB, BS FRCS(E) wishes to research and document the use of Coma Arousal techniques in the severely brain injured and to offer these techniques to those who may wish to use them.

These techniques are still in the process of development and at this stage there is no firm evidence from Australian Sources on their efficiency.

However some reports from the United States indicate that they may be advantageous in reducing the length of Coma and possibly reducing the extent of neurological deficit.

I am satisfied that Dr. Freeman's approach will be ethical and constant.

The Medical Superintendent of the hospital and the Neurosurgeon or Attending medical officer will be first contacted and the matter discussed with them.

Only if they are in agreement and give their permission will the program be explained to the relatives for their involvement.

Dr. Freeman will not intrude in any way, with the control of the patient and the responsibility for the patient will be solely with the patient's medical officer.

Dr. Freeman will work under the authority of that medical officer. Dr. Freeman is not in private practice and no question arises of his treating any patient beyond what is outlined herein.

(The program is non-interventionist from the surgical point of view and consists of intense sensory stimulation.)

It is important that the relatives of the patient should be involved heavily in the program both from the patient's point of view and also to minimise the load on the hospital.

Neither the G.I.O. nor Dr. Freeman makes any specific claims for the technique and it is important that this is understood by all.

However your help and co-operation with Dr. Freeman would be appreciated.

Yours truly,

J. A. Gill
Acting Assistant Managing Director
Government Insurance Office

Two of Sydney's leading neurologists agreed their names could be attached to the research proposal. This automatically meant other professors and doctors in all medical specialties would feel safe in becoming involved, and many also supported the proposed research. The epidemiologist, the psychiatrist and I prepared a research protocol, which was approved by the GIO.

It was important to learn about the management of severe brain injury in other world centres. March 1983 came and Dorothy and I left for overseas. The United States appeared to be the most advanced, although first-rate work had been done in Glasgow. Los Angeles seemed to be a good place to commence but it was disappointing to learn that the International Coma Data Bank, into which I had hoped to incorporate Sydney data, had been discontinued.

My next US contact was in Boston with the US National Head Injury Foundation (NHIF). The NHIF had been started by Marilyn Spivack. Marilyn's daughter had suffered a severe brain injury and Marilyn had become angry with the dismal and negative attitude of the physicians. She directed her energies to joining together families and medical professionals in a productive way. The NHIF produced a newsletter on a regular basis identifying the needs of the patient and the family. Just before my visit to the United States, their *Newsletter* of Spring 1982 contained the words '[i]t is impossible to remain aloof when faced with a family, torn by fright and anger, handicapped by guilt and denial and seemingly abandoned by a system which does not care enough'.

Marilyn started to form chapters of the NHIF in the United States and soon realised that she was not alone in wanting to gather knowledge of the families' predicaments and bring it into mainstream medicine. Within a period of two years, 14 States had formed chapters. It was interesting that even in 1982, Professor Ben Yishay, Associate Professor of Clinical Rehabilitation Medicine at New York University, wrote in the NHIF *Newsletter*:

> I would like to cite the appearance in recent years of several publications which provide us with newer and more hopeful insights into the potential inherent in the human brain for the restoration and reorganisation of functions following brain injury … the traditional model of rehabilitation is not suited for an estimated 80% of persons surviving a traumatic head injury.

While in Boston, I visited a well-known rehabilitation hospital: the Greenery. This was a revelation. It had been opened 10 years previously. There was no morbid feel about the hospital. It was full of US initiative. They had active units that specifically dealt with patients in coma. Vigorous attempts at arousal of the patients took place in an effort to give them every chance to regain function. The Greenery had links with institutions that had high reputations such as Tufts New England Medical Centre and St Elisabeth's Hospital, a teaching affiliate of Tufts University.

My next visit was to the Head Injury Centre at Lewis Bay, Hyannis. This was smaller than the Greenery but had a similar approach. Its Progressive Coma Management Program measured 'the individual's capacity to respond to a variety of sensory inputs', and it admitted patients who had a decreased level of awareness for more than six months—that is, in the persistent vegetative state.

From Boston, I went to the Bronx Municipal Hospital in New York to speak to one of the neurosurgeons. He thought stimulation of the patient in coma was a waste of time. He said that using a torch to give a light input to the eyes would be likely to cause the patient to have an epileptic fit and that the only way the problem could be solved was by developing the chemical transmitters that are used by the brain to send a message from one nerve to another. He was dismissive of any alternatives.

One of my main reasons for going to New York was to make contact with a neurosurgeon, Dr Mihai Dimancescu. Dr Dimancescu had pioneered 'coma stimulation'. He directed the International Coma Recovery Institute in that city. Unfortunately, I could not meet with this great groundbreaking doctor as he had been called away urgently to assess a patient in Europe. Some years later we did meet and shared our experiences.

On the Sunday when we were in New York we went to church in the lovely, historical Fifth Avenue Presbyterian Church. It was special for us because the choir sang Gabriel Faure's *Requiem*, which starts with: 'Grant them rest eternal, O Lord, and let light perpetual shine on them.' The minister who conducted the funeral service for our son Matthew had told us that on the night after the funeral he had sung this *Requiem* with a major Sydney choral group.

I had seen enough in the United States to support a new approach to coma. It seemed that much was already being done in the United States. I could not foresee that there would be any difficulty in introducing such an approach into the hospitals and the medical profession in Australia. I had not, however, taken into consideration the massive power base that would be required to achieve any shift in the present treatment of coma; I should have known better.

The epidemiologist, the psychiatrist and I realised that the protocol for the coma arousal research must be undertaken in a major Australian hospital. Soon after my return to Australia, we approached the neurosurgeons at Royal North Shore Hospital and Westmead Hospital and presented the protocol to them, accompanied by the letter from GIO. They showed some reserve, but were not opposed to the further development of the document. One of them said that 'anything which can be done to help these victims of brain injury would be welcomed'.

By June 1983, the protocol had gained wide support from the universities and hospitals in Sydney. Kevin Beckton expressed GIO's pleasure at its progress. While both Royal North Shore and Westmead hospitals had been approached initially, Westmead, a large hospital in western Sydney with an excellent reputation, seemed to be the more receptive. What's more, Westmead needed a piece of equipment for research. They were $20 000 short of the money needed.

Kevin Beckton agreed that GIO would donate this amount. Westmead was also better for me personally since I knew some of the doctors from student days at medical school. I studied intensely everything in the medical journals that related to coma and brain injury. There was a lot of activity in overseas centres: in the United States at Richmond, Virginia, and also in Britain at London and Glasgow. The developed countries were now recognising that brain injury had reached epidemic proportions and was a massive problem.[12]

By the end of 1983 the protocol had been scrutinised and passed by the Ethics and Research committees of the Westmead Hospital, and the GIO decided to fund a feasibility study on coma arousal at Westmead Hospital. Kevin Beckton notified me that he had received permission from the GIO Board to provide research finance that would allow clinical research to commence at Westmead. The research protocol required the cooperation of many different departments in Westmead. These included neurology, neurosurgery, intensive care, rehabilitation, nursing, social work, physiotherapy, occupational therapy and speech pathology. Each department was autonomous, but interlocked, and each needed to be encouraged to take part. The Director of Research Resources at the hospital told me that the hospital had never had such a large research proposal before.

Conclusion

Ted Freeman's account of his life preceding a commitment to people with brain injury identifies events that afforded him insights into the experiences of those people and their families. Coupled with this was the horror evoked in him, and others, by the conditions in which many people with severe, long-term disabilities were maintained within the healthcare system. A possible solution to some of his concerns was offered by the availability, from a large insurance company, of financial support to research the possibilities for improvements to the existing situation.

---

12   Bryan Jennett & Graham Teasdale (1977) Aspects of coma after severe head injury. *The Lancet, 1*, 78.

2. Misdiagnosis: Patients' stories

Statistics of brain injuries cannot adequately convey their longer-term impact on affected people and certainly fail to reveal the manner in which decisions and commitments made, on their behalf by others, can influence their longer-term outcomes. This chapter examines the stories of 10 of Ted Freeman's patients, based on his clinical notes and written by him so as to facilitate their accessibility to lay readers. These stories are reproduced without modification and have been selected from two dozen included by Freeman in a chronological account of his work. That selection has been undertaken in order to illustrate a number of recurrent features.

One recurrent feature is that of an inaccurate early diagnosis of vegetative state. Although the international medical literature had repeatedly drawn attention to the frequency of incorrect diagnosis of vegetative states, this caution does not seem to have been understood. Faulty diagnosis led to the formulation of a prognosis that was invariably very negative. That prognosis, in its turn, was liable to lead to a management recommendation that the patient was unsuitable for formal rehabilitation and should receive no more than basic care. In the ensuing months and years, the ultimate condition of some patients and, with it, any potential for later improvement were further compromised as a direct outcome of the recommendation.

The total number of people with severe brain injuries whom Freeman was asked to see in the course of his career amounted to approximately 200. Whereas a majority of these became long-term patients, some were assessed only once. In relation to the latter group, Freeman explained that they

> tended to be patients who were unresponsive and it appeared that attempting to impose a program that was demanding and impossible to fulfil on the family would have stressed them beyond reason. I had to be honest with the family and tell them that I did not think I could help.

In some instances, the diagnosis of 'vegetative' was patently wrong at the time that Freeman met the patient; in others, it subsequently ceased to be applicable. The term 'vegetative state' is applied when a patient periodically has open eyes but, nevertheless, is considered to be unconscious. Alternatively, if the patient's eyes remain closed, the condition is described as 'coma'. Since then, the adoption of 'vegetative' as a term in popular parlance has very successfully corrupted its meaning. For example, referees at football matches are commonly denigrated as 'vegetative' and the adjective has spawned its corresponding verb: one may now 'veg out' in front of a television set. Unfortunately, this popular loose application appears often to have re-entered medical use. One suspects that it has frequently been thrown around without the completion of thorough, repeated clinical examinations.

The first two of Freeman's case reports exemplify either initial misdiagnosis (Peter) or premature and unduly pessimistic diagnosis (Donald). In these, as in all of the following case histories, patients' names have been altered. Of particular concern in Donald's case, as remarked in Freeman's notes, was the reference by the attending registrar to 'brain death'. As the question of organ donation had been broached with the family, the possibility that one or more of the people attending Donald had made a formal (mis)diagnosis seems credible.

As with the term 'vegetative', the expression 'brain death' has acquired a life outside intensive care wards—again, sports referees are often categorised as brain dead. It would be most unfortunate if this term has also crept back into some hospitals in its imprecise use. Accounts given by families of severely brain injured patients refer to 'vegetative' quite often; less frequently to 'brain death' with discussion of organ donation. As the original source of these references when they arise in families' accounts at a later stage cannot be retrospectively verified, it is not usually practicable to differentiate misinforming of relatives from inaccurate recollection. The excuse of impaired family recollection is not applicable in the case of Donald, which follows.

Donald's story

I saw Donald in a major teaching hospital. His sister had asked me to assess him. I went to see the Medical Superintendent first. She did not approve of my involvement, but gave me permission to see Donald. I spoke to the Neurosurgical Registrar. He told me that there was no point in seeing Donald, saying he was 'brain dead'. His family had been asked to donate his organs. I met Donald's wife and sister, who took me to examine Donald. I could not detect any positive reactions. I told them so. I suggested that a trial of 'coma arousal therapy' might be warranted. The family agreed.

That night Donald's sister rang and asked what I intended to do. I explained that I could not return to the hospital—I would be refused entry. She was a courageous lady. She said, 'That's not good enough. Will you come and tell us what to do?' Two days later I went to their house in a Sydney suburb and told them what I thought could be done. I discussed a coma arousal program with them and they wrote it down.

I heard no more for some weeks until Donald's sister, only a very tiny lady but obviously very determined, rang me. She said, 'I know you are not going to believe this, Dr Freeman. We did everything you told us to do every day. I went in there today and worked on him and said to him, "Donald, we come here and work on you all day long and you never say anything."' She continued: 'He slowly turned his head towards me and said "Hello".' I was amazed. Donald was eventually sent to a rehabilitation hospital and later returned home, where I saw him again. He talked clearly and lucidly, walked with a walking stick, fed himself and possessed bowel and bladder control. He has since successfully completed a technical course.

This story has a worrying aspect. It casts doubt on the diagnosis of brain death, but clarification would be needed as to whether a neurosurgeon gave this diagnosis. I have seen two other patients whose families told me the person was considered brain dead. One patient did remarkably well and is walking and talking and driving his four-wheel drive on holidays with his family. The other is still slowly improving.

Peter's story

On another occasion I was asked to assess Peter. He had been placed in a terminal-care hospital for people who had suffered a stroke or had end-stage cancer. Peter was in his early forties. Once again the diagnosis was 'vegetative'. I waited for a family member to come, but as none was available I commenced the assessment. I knew as soon as I met Peter that he was aware. He made eye contact immediately. I said to him, 'Peter, I know you can understand everything I say to you. Would you blink both eyes for me?' He did so. I asked, 'Will you blink your left eye?' He did so. 'Will you raise both thumbs?' He complied. 'Will you raise your right thumb first and then your left thumb?' He did so. I asked him to move his legs. He did. I was very excited. This man was demonstrably capable of understanding and complying with many requests. The diagnosis was absolutely wrong and could easily be shown to be so. I left the room and found the Nurse Unit Manager. I told her what I had found and asked her to come back to the room and observe with me. She hesitated, but agreed to do so. With encouragement, Peter showed his range of abilities again.

I telephoned Peter's referring doctor and gave him a description of what I had found. He showed no interest. I was distraught and unsure what to do. I asked his permission to speak to Peter's relatives. He agreed grudgingly. He clearly resented my interference. My heart sank when the nurse brought in a lady in her late sixties already in grief and of non-Australian background and I went out to the nurse and asked for other relatives. There were none. I told her I would make a detailed report of my finding and send it to the doctor. I went back to the room to say goodbye to Peter. His mother was sitting by his bedside weeping over him. I left, feeling almost as distressed as his mother. The following day I prepared a detailed report and posted it immediately to Peter's doctor. He did not acknowledge it. One week later I rang the doctor to check to make sure he had received my report. I said, 'This is

Ted Freeman. I am just ringing to make sure you have my medical report on Peter. How is he?' He replied: 'Thanks for the report, Dr Freeman. Peter died two days ago.' I was stunned. 'What did he die from?' I asked. 'He had a severe attack of diarrhoea and we thought in view of his severe brain injury we would not treat him.' I exclaimed, 'But he had so much that could have been worked on and such potential!' He replied, 'We did not think so.' I said, 'So he died from dehydration and electrolyte imbalance?' He said, 'That is correct.' I put the phone down in dismay.

Misdiagnosis: Implications for treatment

Apart from their common feature of a misleading diagnosis and subsequent prognosis, the stories of Donald and Peter illustrate some other incidents frequently occurring in Freeman's case records. Not uncommonly, treatment was withheld from patients considered to be vegetative at an early stage after injury because, in the opinion of the treating practitioners, future quality of life would be sufficiently poor that its occurrence was best avoided. This does raise the question of the time frame after brain injury for diagnosis of the vegetative state.

There is no ethical imperative to provide treatment irrespective of its intensity or invasiveness and of the patient's potential for achieving an improved quality of life. Any reasonable application of the concept of proportionality would rely upon some balancing between the possible discomfort to be inflicted on the patient by treatment and the quantum of possible benefit. 'Extraordinary' measures (however one defines them) may well not have been appropriate in Peter's case, but what appears to have been forgone (probably intravenous fluids and antibiotics) could hardly be dismissed as 'extraordinary' in assessment of a patient who evinced considerable (unrecognised) potential for improvement.

As a general principle, or perhaps a general lack of principle, Peter's case seems to have been an example of medical opportunism in which 'routine' treatment, unlikely to be uncomfortable for the patient, is withheld *because* that course of action is likely to lead to death. When the alternatives of non-intervention *versus* the 'Freeman' approach intended to offer the best chance of regaining consciousness are discussed in a later chapter, this point will be taken up again. There is also a 'third way'—namely, withdrawing medical support at an early stage, thereby precluding any determination of what potential for improvement could have existed.

Another aspect of these two cases that should be noted here, although its more detailed discussion will also be deferred, was the rejection by his colleagues of any involvement by Freeman in these cases. As will be described in Chapter 7, he was told not to return to Donald by the Neurosurgical Registrar: his report on Peter was unacknowledged and discounted by the general practitioner.

The outcome in Peter's case contrasts sharply with that of any of the patients to be discussed in the next chapter. That chapter will discuss a few of the stories of the families of young people with very severe brain injuries. Most of these people had fewer early signs of regained awareness than Peter and, for this reason, might have been considered less likely ultimately to achieve favourable outcomes. They differed from Peter, however, in having families who were prepared to do whatever might offer some hope of improving the lot of their brain injured family member. As will be recounted in that chapter, these relatives regularly resisted advice to abandon the person and instead committed the family to a prolonged domiciliary rehabilitation program that made enormous demands on them. It does not require too much reflection on these stories to recognise that the best prognostic feature predisposing to recovery after comparable degrees of injury is to have such a family. Peter, unfortunately, did not.

Whereas the stories of Donald and Peter were chosen to illustrate the tendency for a diagnosis of 'vegetative' to be applied loosely, and frequently inaccurately, the next two stories illustrate some of the early consequences of this common tendency.

Misdiagnosis: Ethical considerations

Roger's story

As Ted Freeman wrote:

The phone rang early one morning at home just as I was about to leave for work at Peat Island. A father asked me to assess his son Roger. Roger, who was eighteen, had been riding his motorbike down a bush track two years before. An unknown person had strung a wire between two trees at shoulder height. It caught Roger around the throat, smashed his windpipe and knocked him off his bike. He stopped breathing for some minutes and his brain became damaged due to lack of oxygen. 'What can he do?' I asked. 'He can't do anything. We have been told that he is a vegetable. They call him persistent vegetative state,'[1] the father replied.

I drove to their farmhouse. Roger's father met me at the front door. We shook hands and I walked in to meet his wife. I followed them into the family room

---

1 Bryan Jennett & Fred Plum (1972) Persistent vegetative state after brain damage. A syndrome in search of a name. *The Lancet, i*, 734.

where the patient lay motionless on his back, stretched out full length on a brown leather, padded bench. It was hot in the house. He had one sheet under him and one covering him. His eyes were closed. I walked over with his father, stood at his right side and introduced myself. 'Roger, my name is Ted Freeman. I am a doctor. Your mother and father have asked me to come to see you.' There was no movement, no speech, no facial expression or reaction. He remained motionless. I noted both pupils were widely dilated (enlarged)—a sign of damage to both oculomotor nerves in the mid-brain region of the brainstem. I carried out a neurological examination that confirmed he had severe brain injury.

I asked Roger's father, 'Can Roger do anything?' He pulled out a small object and said, 'Not much. One thing he will do is reach for this cartridge [a shiny brass army bullet casing]. Roger can see, but he cannot hold his eyes open. I have been told the nerves to his eyelids have been damaged.' With his thumb and the index finger of his left hand, the father prised both his son's upper eyelids open. The father took the cartridge in his right hand and held it above Roger's face. Slowly, he raised the cartridge and said to his son, 'Take this shell.' Little by little, Roger's right hand moved up until his fingers closed on the shell and he took it.

The parents had been told that this young man was in the persistent vegetative state (PVS). The diagnosis was obviously wrong. Roger was not vegetative. He was a thinking human being with the ability to hear and understand the spoken word and the motor skill to move his right hand and arm towards an object and grasp it with his fingers. They said that 'the lights are on but no-one is at home'. I asked, 'What else can he do?' The father replied, 'I can get him to cry.' Before I could stop him, he moved to a record player, switched it on and said, 'This record always makes him cry!' The music was the recent recording of a pop group. When the music started, Roger started to sob loudly. Tears flowed over his cheeks wetting the sheet under him. I asked the father to stop the record and said, 'This is more proof that your son is not vegetative. He can feel emotions. He can think and he has memory. This means his higher brain is working. He is in the "locked-in state".'[2]

What can be more terrifying than to be absolutely at the mercy of your environment and the people in it, and totally unable to control what happens to you? Some patients can be observed by their families or nursing and other healthcare professionals to demonstrate awareness and therefore cannot be considered as PVS. They are in the 'locked-in state'. I call this state the 'ultimate dungeon'. These unfortunate people have a brain that has the ability to process the stimuli from the environment through their eyes, ears, skin, taste and smell, and so on, but their brain stem has been damaged so much that they cannot work their muscles or use speech to communicate to others. There has been recognition of this dilemma for some years.

---

2   Jean-Dominique Bauby (1997) *The Diving Bell and the Butterfly.* Fourth Estate, London.

How could Roger be diagnosed as in coma or vegetative when he was so obviously aware? Second, why was it that the family had observed more than the physicians, and third, why was there no place where Roger could receive treatment? Roger's mother, who had been standing at the back of the room watching, walked over to her son and put her arms around him. Crying, she turned to her husband and said, 'I knew they were wrong. I knew they were wrong, but you would not listen to me.' I had seen this situation before. I spoke to both parents. 'This wrong diagnosis is not your fault. It happens commonly with patients like Roger. There are some members of the medical profession who declare people as PVS without really examining them properly and at a far too early time frame after the injury.'

Roger's parents stared at me. 'What can we do? Can you help?' they asked. We sat down with a cup of tea and explored the options. There were not many. Roger had already been discharged from the teaching hospital and had been ruled as 'not suitable for rehabilitation' by the rehabilitation service.

Most doctors they had spoken to about the continuing treatment of brain injury had told them nothing could be done with these people. The common attitude was the one held by the medical superintendent of a large Australian institution for disabled people. He believed, and I quote: 'The hardest single aspect of coping with head injuries is that fundamentally we are all spectators as the recovery process takes place.' Of course, if we can only observe the process of recovery and not take an active part, there is no point in having rehabilitation units.

Roger's parents were grateful when I had him admitted into a terminal-care hospital that had a minor rehabilitation component. There he came under the care of a doctor with the typical negative approach to these patients. Roger was given no rehabilitation. The admission became one of respite care for his parents. In fairness to the hospital, they were chronically short of nursing and paramedical staff. Roger was no trouble for the hospital to look after. A patient who cannot speak or move but lies in bed or sits strapped in a wheelchair all day does not require much nursing care apart from attention to food, bowels and bladder. Oral feeding, which may be carried out at home by family members, is often dispensed with in the hospital and replaced with a tube into the stomach through which semi-fluid nutrients are fed. This is far less time-consuming than feeding a person with a spoon mouthful by mouthful; but it denies the patient the pleasure of taste—one of life's delights. You don't have to be a gourmet to enjoy food.

Since Roger could not open his eyes, he enjoyed listening to his music from audio tapes. So that he would not disturb the other patients, he listened through headphones. These had to be placed in position by the nursing staff. One day Roger's father brought him audio tapes that contained some erotic dialogue. Roger enjoyed these immensely. He smiled and laughed and the erotic stimulation produced a penile erection. A member of the nursing staff became suspicious when she saw Roger's reactions to his tapes. She put on the headphones and listened. What she heard disturbed her greatly. She reported this matter to the Director of Nursing, who regarded the whole matter as unseemly. The tapes were removed from this young man and the parents were told that if they wanted him to listen to 'that disgusting stuff' they would have to take him home. They were in a quandary. They made the decision to take him home so they could care for him again. I saw him at home again, but four months later he died from asphyxiation after inhaling food. This couple had had two sons. Their eldest had died some years before.

There is something dramatically wrong with a scientific or medical system that condemns people to a life worse than death when knowledge that could help has been available for decades. This is not just a medical issue. It must be one of the major ethical and moral issues of our time.

Rupe's story

Rupe was a patient I examined about four weeks after his injury. He was a man in his early forties who had been diagnosed as vegetative. His wife, Aileen met me at the terminal-care hospital. She was very supportive of her husband. After I had talked for some time to Aileen, she took me to Rupe's bedside. It was immediately clear to me that Rupe was not vegetative. He was able to obey numerous commands and he demonstrated a great deal of awareness. Aileen was delighted to observe his responses as all the information so far that had been given to her had been that Rupe was vegetative and his prognosis poor. She could see for herself that he was recovering. I recommended that Rupe be transferred as rapidly as possible to a rehabilitation hospital. I left the hospital in high spirits, elated by the fact that this man could be saved. I heard no more about this patient until three years later. Aileen phoned me and asked if I would see Rupe, who was now in a nursing home. 'What has happened?' I asked. The whole sorry story of neglect then came out. He had not been given enough time to respond well at the rehabilitation hospital, in fact only a few months, and then the insurance company had transferred him to a nursing home.

I introduced myself. 'I am Ted Freeman. I am a doctor. I have seen you before, some years ago. Is it all right if I examine you?' He ignored me. Instead, his right hand went to the Communicator machine and by the use of his index finger he commenced to punch some letters into the machine. I could not see what he was writing, but when he had finished he punched another key and the message was spoken. 'Have you been to medical school?' I laughed and replied, 'Yes, I have. You need have no worries about that.' He looked at me again and turned to punch out another message on his Communicator. I waited, wondering what it would be.

He finished typing and pressed his voice activator to broadcast, 'I don't want any mug looking after me!'

Rupe and I got on well. The nursing home was receptive and keen to help so we soon had Rupe standing on one leg and pulling himself out of his chair. He was much happier and he knew that he was slowly regaining some function. Aileen was very pleased, but one day all therapy was stopped. The nursing home expressed concern that Rupe might fall or that the nurses could hurt their backs. There was no such thing as the 'dignity of risk' for Rupe. Rupe did have a legal case against the insurance company. He was an innocent party in the accident and his case came up in the Supreme Court in another State in a major provincial city. I had done numerous medico-legal reports for the barristers representing Rupe. They were going to fly Rupe and Aileen to the city where his case was to be heard. They asked me if I would be prepared to give evidence in the Supreme Court. I agreed. I arrived the day after Rupe and Aileen. Aileen told me that the previous night, she had taken Rupe to the casino and he had had a 'wow of a time' on the 'pokies', and so on. The morning of the court case he met the policeman who had pulled him from the burning wreckage of his vehicle. Rupe had cried and constantly typed out on his Communicator, 'Thank you. Thank you. Thank you.'

When I arrived at the court the barristers asked me if I could demonstrate the extent of Rupe's cognitive function to the judge. They said they would move Rupe into the court early so that he could become accustomed to the atmosphere. Rupe's wheelchair was pushed to the front of the courtroom. There he sat twisted and bent and all scrunched up with his Communicator on his knee. The court reporters were watching him closely, wondering what was happening as Rupe sat tapping away with one finger at his Communicator. I became worried. Would he make some inappropriate statement that would be broadcast over the whole of the court and be prejudicial to his case? After some minutes, the court official entered and in a loud voice called, 'Silence, please. All rise. In the name of Her Majesty Queen Elizabeth. This court is now in session.' His honour the judge entered. All rose to their feet and bowed—that is, all except Rupe. At that precise moment, he pressed his audio button and the words rang out loudly and clearly around the Supreme Court, repeating: 'I hope the judge will forgive me for not standing. I hope the judge will forgive me for not standing. I hope the judge will forgive me for not standing.'

At first the judge was taken aback by this unusual occurrence. He looked towards Rupe. The moment he acknowledged Rupe's request, Rupe stopped his message. He was not perseverating at all. He only wished to be acknowledged as a human being. It was easy to present the evidence for medical misdiagnosis. In fact, it was a 'lay-down misère'! The judgment was made in favour of Rupe and against the insurance company. In my opinion, the question must be asked why this man was cast into this horrendous predicament.

Roger and Rupe represent two more instances of misdiagnosis of vegetative state. In Rupe's case, this error should have been immediately evident any time that he was examined, and the question posed by Ted Freeman of why he was cast into such a horrendous predicament is entirely appropriate. Recognition that Roger was not vegetative was not so immediately apparent and it is easy to understand how a conventional neurological examination could get it wrong, especially if the clinician was not endowed with good interpersonal skills.

In the absence of the regular Freeman approach of recruiting a family member or close friend when setting out to examine a patient, the information that Roger regularly responded to certain specific stimuli, and hence the occurrence of these responses, could not have been elicited. Whilst operating through a family member was Freeman's regular practice, intended to place a patient at ease, in Roger's case it delivered a bonus of information. I am inclined to add a postscript to the quotation from a medical superintendent referring to patients with severe brain injuries and cited by Freeman—perhaps it should be: 'we are all spectators *and often not very careful ones.*'

Apart from sharing the misfortune of misdiagnosis, Roger and Rupe illustrate the manner in which this primary event can lead to system-mediated deprivation. In Roger's case, the opportunity to receive auditory input through his headphones was taken away. His tears on the occasion of Ted Freeman's initial examination and his arousal in response to a tape recording when in the nursing home indicated not only a level of consciousness, but also a capacity for emotional response—an even more damning refutation of a 'vegetative' diagnosis. Further sensory deprivation is likely to have been imposed by the replacement of oral feeding, with its attendant sensations of taste, texture and scent, with tube feeding. In Rupe's case, the sentence imposed by the system was three years in a nursing home after a short attempt at rehabilitation. Even some well-intentioned small attempts at rehabilitation were aborted because of possible 'risk' (one wonders whether only to the patient or also to the system to which he had been committed).

Roger was a person who was 'locked in' as a direct result of his brain injury. While his ability to see things and to hear and understand conversations remained intact, he had extremely limited ability to undertake actions in response, which would have confirmed that he was aware and could see, hear and comprehend. In very severe cases of being 'locked in', a person may be completely aware but restricted to using nothing more than eye movements to respond.

Cecil's story: Locked in by the system

In contrast with being locked in because of damage to those parts of the brain required to respond, some of Freeman's patients could be appropriately regarded as locked in by the system in which they were placed. Cecil, whose story follows, provides an example of such a predicament.

Cecil had been a fit young man, married with a family, when he had a motor vehicle accident and was severely brain injured. The care he received in the emergency department and operating theatres, I assume, was excellent for he had been admitted to a major Sydney teaching hospital, which had a superb reputation. As well as his brain injury he had broken bones: fractures of his left humerus (upper arm) and right femur (upper leg). Because of the extent of his brain injury, it was decided not to operate but to treat his fractures 'conservatively'. That means to put his arm in a sling and possibly to splint his right leg. (The usual treatment of such injuries would be to operate and fix the broken bones in place by means of plates or pins, and so on.) Three months after his accident, Cecil was transferred to a terminal-care hospital with the diagnosis of 'vegetative state', and six months after the injury he was assessed by a rehabilitation specialist, who wrote: 'In view of his cerebral cortical damage, his semi rigid limbs with contractures and the length of time since the injury, I would not advocate rehabilitative procedures and would urge consideration not to treat infections with antibiotics.'

Eight months after Cecil's accident, his father asked me to assess his son. I asked if members of the family could be present, but was told that this was not possible. His wife did not want the assessment. On the prearranged day, I presented myself to the Director of Nursing, who gave me the clinical notes. She escorted me to the ward. There were six beds in the ward. The room was dark and smelt of human decay. I thanked the director, who retired. I approached Cecil and drew up a chair next to his bed so I was at his eye level. I did not want to stand over him. He immediately made eye contact and looked at me directly as I explained who I was and why I was there. I told him that I would not hurt him and that every time I intended to touch him I would tell him. He continued to make excellent eye contact. In fact, his eyes were glued to my face. I spoke openly to him. I placed my hand in his right hand and asked him to squeeze it. He grasped it strongly. There is a 'grasp reflex' in many people with a severe brain injury, which occurs instantly you put something into their hand. This is similar to the reflex action of an infant when an object is placed into his or her hand. I asked Cecil to release his grip. He did so immediately. The release of the grasp indicated this was not a reflex happening but an active movement with the muscles controlled by the brain.

I held a torch in front of Cecil's face and moved it from side to side and asked him to follow it with his eyes. He did so. I shifted it further to the right and asked him to turn his head so he could see it. He did so. He did the same when I placed it on his left side. I asked Cecil for permission to examine his arms and legs. He nodded his head in agreement. His left arm and right leg had united in an abnormal position. I asked him if I could feel the fracture sites. He nodded. I did so and it was obvious he had no pain. I asked him to move his left leg and straighten it out. He did so. I said to him, 'Cecil, I know that you can understand everything I say to you. If you believe this to be true, can you nod your head.' He nodded his head several times.

I realised I was the first person to show Cecil that I knew he was out of coma and it was important I tell him of this fact and that I would do all I could to help him. As I did so, tears came into his eyes. I said goodbye, and put out my hand to shake hands. He slowly reached out with his right hand and attempted to take mine and shake it.

I left the ward and went to the nurses' station and spoke to some of the nursing staff. They agreed that Cecil showed emotion. 'When is the most emotion you have seen?' I asked. They replied as one: 'When his wife brings in his children, he always cries!' This confirmed my findings. This man was not in PVS. He wasn't even severely locked in. He had loads of comprehension and a great deal of movement, which I believed could be increased with therapy—enough to free him from his dungeon. I rang Cecil's doctor and told him my conclusions and the evidence upon which they were based. He appeared disinterested. I asked if I could make contact with Cecil's wife. He said she had been told her husband was vegetative and to go away and forget all about him. I persevered. 'Okay,' he said. 'I will see if she will agree to meet with you. Give me your phone number.'

Some days later, Cecil's wife rang me. 'What is the point of a meeting?' she asked. I explained my findings to her. 'I don't think that changes anything. I have been told nothing can be done,' she replied. I pushed for a meeting. Eventually, she came to the terminal-care hospital to meet me. It was a great disappointment. I asked her to walk with me into Cecil's room so I could demonstrate Cecil's awareness and my findings. She refused. I suggested that we arrange a 'trial of rehabilitation therapy' for Cecil. She refused. She said, 'I just want my husband to be kept comfortable.' How she believed keeping Cecil in his present state would provide mental and emotional comfort for him I could not understand. I could do nothing more. I was powerless to help Cecil. I wrote out a detailed clinical report and sent it to Cecil's doctor and to his wife and father. I heard no more for some months until Cecil's father asked me to review his son again.

By this time Cecil had been assessed again by the rehabilitation specialist, 11 months after the accident. He wrote:

> *The patient has changed a little. He can now lift a cup with his left thumb and forefinger and drink. He sometimes indicates 'yes' and 'no' with minuscule neck movements appropriately but not often. I do not consider any form of rehabilitation or stimulation therapy is indicated.*

It was obvious that this doctor had a very negative approach, but even he must have known that the obeying of a command was a prime indication of the patient being out of coma or PVS. He advocated transfer to a nursing home. When Cecil's father contacted me again he was distraught. Not only had he and his wife lost their son, but now friction had developed with his daughter-in-law over Cecil's treatment. The intensity of the emotion meant they were denied contact with their grandchildren.

Fifteen months after the accident, Cecil was moved to a nursing home. I heard no more of this man during this time. Two years and four months after the accident, Cecil was assessed by a psychiatrist, who noted the opinion of a nursing sister. She was emphatic that the patient was largely aware of what was going on. If he did not like a TV program, he shook his head. If he did not like a particular activity, he would stiffen and close his eyes. He appeared to enjoy the visits of his children and on one occasion wept when told they were away on holidays and would not be there. In summary, the psychiatrist stated:

> *The fact that he does communicate indicates a greater degree of awareness of his surroundings than was originally thought possible … It is probable that he also has some awareness of the major changes in his mental and physical state and that he does, in fact, suffer as a result.*

At much the same time, a report was prepared by an orthopaedic surgeon, who noted: 'All his fractures united though not in a position which would have been considered acceptable for an otherwise well patient.'

Cecil's left arm was now 3 cm shorter than the other and his right leg was 6 cm shorter than his left. Both fractures had united with overlapping, separation and angulation. I had no further contact with the patient until four years after his accident when I examined him in the nursing home. He obeyed many commands. Once again, I urged in my report that '[e]very effort should be made for him to regain, by urgent and intensive rehabilitation, more adequate means of communication'. Nothing was done. Two years after this (six years post accident), he was admitted to a rehabilitation hospital for two weeks. They reported:

> *He was able to assist with transfers. He was generally uncooperative with therapy tasks and this would appear to mitigate against future gains. It is recommended that a much longer trial of speech therapy assessment would be needed … in order to more accurately assess his potential.*

As you can imagine, two weeks of therapy after a delay of six years can only be described as absurd. He could assist with transferring from a chair to a bed or vice versa so he was able to partially take weight on his left leg, but because he was generally uncooperative they thought that this would be a block on further gains. There was no sensitivity or recognition of the fact that for six years this man, with adequate awareness to comply with requests, had been so hurt mentally, emotionally and physically that he must have had a deep well of anger and frustration eating away inside him—enough to make him uncooperative. But having lost all control over his environment, this in the end was the only way he could exert his willpower. Perhaps if someone had asked him what he wanted to do rather than telling him what to do, he might have been more cooperative.

I have always been a strong believer that the anger and aggression in a person with a brain injury are their body language indicating that they do not like their present situation or what has happened to them. I am a firm believer that if this anger is worked with and is channelled correctly, it has the potential to be extremely productive. If, instead, the patient is damped down with drugs or is physically restrained with belts and straps to the bed or chair, the frustration and anger will only increase.

Cecil's parents were distraught with the system that had done this to their son. They could see Cecil was aware and in a terrible plight. They asked to meet with me to discuss what could be done to help him. Seven years after Cecil's accident, I was asked to review Cecil again in the nursing home. I went through the usual protocol and, having been given permission, went to his room. He immediately turned his eyes and head towards me.

I said 'hello' and put out my hand to him. He did not shake hands. He was about to have some morning tea, which consisted of a glass of flavoured milk and some fruitcake. I asked him which he would like first. He nodded towards the milk. I asked him if I could sit and talk to him, and also did he remember me. He nodded 'yes' to both. After his morning tea I asked him to move his head, arms, hands, fingers and legs, and he happily complied with my requests. When I asked him if he could stand, he nodded 'yes' and, with me supporting him, he stood on his left leg. His right leg was shortened and could not touch the floor. After an hour or so, I thanked him for his attention and went and spoke to the nursing staff. They said that he was receiving one hour of therapy per week and had not been taken home for some years. They said he often wrestled with them and had on occasions tried to kick them. I explained to them that this aggressive behaviour was his body language stating emphatically that he was most unhappy about his situation. It was a perfectly normal reaction to his unresolved predicament. They said he often sat crying.

I wrote to his doctor:

> *Because of his [Cecil's] great awareness of the environment and his very significant emotional response, I consider he is in a state of great sensory and emotional deprivation which constitutes a grave disadvantage to him. To maintain this patient in the present circumstances, without him being given the opportunity to prove his ability to regain function is medically and morally unacceptable.*

I proposed a plan of management. The doctor failed to acknowledge my report.

I did see Cecil at one more nursing home. I was delighted when the Director of Nursing asked me if I would be prepared to give a lecture to the staff and readily agreed. The nursing staff divided rapidly into two groups. There were those who were amused by Cecil's behaviour and regarded him as a bit of a joke. These people were not interested in seeing the humanity in Cecil. There was another group led by a senior nurse who said that she often gave Cecil a cuddle and he would respond by clinging onto her and reacted to her caressing and patting. This nurse provided the only sensitive touch that Cecil received, as his wife and children never visited him. His parents, because of their age, had now become incapable of travelling to the nursing home to support him.

Soon after this I was notified by the Director of Nursing that Cecil's wife said she would prefer I did not see him again as my visits upset Cecil too much. I had to comply with this request, but I believe Cecil realised he had potential to progress and became angry when this was not recognised by the nursing staff.

Cecil concurrently sustained fractures of his arm and leg in the accident responsible for his brain injury. His clinical history when Ted Freeman first met him eight months after that accident described his early orthopaedic management as 'conservative'. Given the detail of what had been done, or more accurately what had not been done, the euphemism 'conservative' should have read 'limited to first aid'. Whereas some of the patients whose stories have been included above developed contractures and stiffening of limbs as a consequence of subsequent neglect in management (euphemistically reported in case notes as 'unsuitable for rehabilitation'), Cecil's subsequent deformities were completely predictable, given the withholding of routine orthopaedic treatment, and completely attributable to that withholding. The withholding reflected an assessment that was based on premature and incorrect prediction of his capacity for neurological recovery, on an erroneous assessment of his conscious state in the weeks after his accident, or both.

As a result of the early decision not to provide any treatment worthy of the name for his fractures and of unwillingness on the part of his medical attendants to reverse that decision later, Cecil was effectively locked in by his mobility limitations. As Freeman remarked in his notes at his first meeting with Cecil, he was the first person to tell Cecil that he knew he was out of coma. In response to the ongoing belief of others that he was unaware of events around him, Cecil was subjected to ongoing sensory and emotional deprivation, presumably for the remainder of his life.

His misery was further compounded by the intra-family disruption between his parents and his wife, an event to which his medical management had in no small way contributed. His wife accepted and acted upon the medical advice that Cecil was vegetative and she should go away and forget about him. His parents resembled most of the families of other people who sought Freeman's advice in not accepting this 'solution'. It appears to me to be self-evident that any other people with severe brain injury whose relatives accepted the negative prognosis that they were given, as did Cecil's wife, would not show up in any review of long-term outcomes. In effect, they would become an unquantifiable cohort similar to the family of Peter, referred to above, when life-sustaining measures had been withdrawn, on the basis of a misdiagnosed 'vegetative state'.

Domiciliary programs

One of the criticisms of the implementation of domiciliary programs to assist people with long-term brain injury is that this option may place great strains on family interactions. As will be seen when families' stories are presented in the next chapter, this is certainly possible. To introduce some context, however, I believe that this is at least as likely to eventuate under a policy of 'go away and forget', but published studies on the families of this more compliant group do not appear to exist. Freeman's closing reflection that Cecil's parents were 'distraught with the system that had done this to their son' provides a fitting epilogue to his story. Whilst the term 'locked in' when applied in relation to the medical condition of a patient with brain injury is taken to refer exclusively to disablement attributable to that injury, the preceding stories illustrate the manner in which a patient's disability can be greatly augmented by inappropriate management. In effect, a patient may be locked in by the system.

Recovery: Patients' stories

Contrasting with the rather dismal stories of Peter, Roger, Rupe and Cecil in which each of these patients' potential for improvement was curtailed for a variety of reasons, in many other instances, this potential was realised. An essential factor in achieving this difference was the nature of family responses to the diagnoses and accompanying prognoses. These responses shared a common feature—namely, not to accept the proposition that nothing could be done to assist their family member.

This chapter will conclude with five of Freeman's case histories recounting instances in which families resolved to do everything in their power. All five people were the subject of dismal prognoses. All five were taken home. All achieved vastly more than had been foreshadowed while they were residents of institutions, albeit the ultimate levels of recovery within the group varied considerably. All expressed pleasure in being alive notwithstanding their various limitations. Yet, as will become apparent from their case histories, all differed in many aspects of that recovery. It is not valid to assume that the damage produced in the brain of any two patients is identical and, consequently, one can never assert with certainty that differences in outcome are unequivocally a reflection of differences in management. That said, it is very likely that the much better outcomes in the remaining patients owe much to the commitment of their families.

Mark's story: Family therapy

Mark was in a country hospital. His parents, Roy and June, were desperately anxious to help their son. They had been told that Mark's case was 'hopeless'. They were told he had been so severely brain injured that nothing could be done and he should be placed in a nursing home. Mark was covered by third-party accident insurance, but the company disputed responsibility. This doubt about the medical responsibility for Mark's care placed June and Roy in the invidious position of receiving minimal assistance from the normal government healthcare scheme and an unwillingness on the part of the insurance company to provide care. Many carers found themselves in this position, often for many years until the legal matter was resolved.

June and Roy were worried about the time factor and my costs for travelling hundreds of kilometres each way to their town. I settled their anxiety by informing them I would visit Mark without charge to them and would only make a charge against the insurance company if they eventually won their case.

Using Roy and June as my bridge, I went through my assessment protocol, detecting 'soft signs' of awareness. It was obvious that no gain could be made by leaving Mark in hospital, so Roy and June decided to take him home and to work with him with the help of family and friends. Slowly, the benefits of their efforts brought rewards. Mark became very aware, and so a more intense program of movement was started. Mark had a tremor that totally affected his whole body and was very noticeable in his eyes, which flicked constantly to the side.

Slowly, Mark learnt to roll over from his back onto each side, and then to hold his body up on his hands and knees, but he could not move forward. Next he learnt to hold his head and body upright while kneeling with his arms draped over the back of a sturdy armchair. Over the months, he regained more control and, falteringly, he moved one arm forward in an attempt to crawl and with continuing work eventually was able to stand and hold himself upright on his knees. It was a great day when he stood with support. Over the months and years that followed, he relearned to walk with a walking frame. Roy bought a large three-wheel bike for his son and taught him to ride along the streets of his town. No-one could assume that Mark would ever return to his pre-accident state, but his gain is vastly better than being left in a nursing home. Roy and June sent me a letter. They wrote:

I would like to say Ted, we are so proud of Mark. He is doing well. He does not use a manual wheelchair anymore. He walks in a frame. We gave Mark a 40th birthday party and invited 60 of his friends. June and I were so proud of Mark when he stood up and made a speech. It brought tears to our eyes.

Mark's recovery, entailing a slow process of relearning how to raise his body, then to sit up and ultimately to stand, recalls the progress of the growing infant. I doubt that any small child standing for the first time could have received more enthusiastic parental acclamation than Mark received on returning to this milestone. Implicit in his parents' description of his birthday party is the pleasure that he and they experienced in his achievements.

Joe's story: Parental determination

Joe, a jockey, suffered severe brain injury when his horse broke a leg and fell on him. Profound brain injury was diagnosed on his admission to a major city hospital. His father, Kevin, and mother, Audrey, were aghast when told their son was unlikely to survive and, even if he did, he would be vegetative. The hospital proposed disconnecting Joe from his life supports and terminating his life. Kevin met with the hospital administration and challenged the withdrawal of treatment from his son. The hospital said Kevin had little influence in the matter and the power to decide rested with them. Kevin refused to accept their authority and contacted his solicitor to stop the termination of Joe's life. Kevin blocked the hospital's action. Kevin rang me about four months after Joe's accident and asked me to assess Joe in hospital. He was diagnosed as being vegetative. With Kevin present, I assessed Joe. The conditions in which Joe was kept were substandard and the hospital was antagonistic to my presence. They made their feelings known in their general demeanour, and in a very offhand way they provided me with the clinical notes.

Joe's parents were relieved when I told them there was some minor evidence of awareness and they asked anxiously whether I would be prepared to admit him to the Brain Injury Therapy Centre (BITC). I told them I could not give a guarantee that I could help, but if they wished I would admit Joe. Kevin was on tenterhooks as I listened to what he, Audrey and also Joe's sister, Debbie, had observed. Joe arrived at the BITC more aware than when I had assessed him in the hospital. It was obvious that the change of the environment, possibly even the journey, had been beneficial. Dr Ross Fulton assessed him and found him fit to receive the therapy that Kevin gave to his son. Each day Joe improved and this could be measured by the size of the smiles on the faces of Kevin and Audrey. Joe started to communicate 'yes' and 'no' by means of thumb movement—up for 'yes', down for 'no'. Slowly, over the weeks, he held his head up and moved it around to look towards his parents, the staff and the volunteers. With support, he started to sit upright in a chair and reached out with his hands to take objects held in front of him. He was able to move his legs slightly.

He started to swallow and eat. He smiled and laughed at jokes and began to obey commands. He came back into the land of the living. Kevin travelled a 400 km round trip every day to give much of the physical therapy and provide emotional support for Joe. After five months at the centre, Joe was taken home and the program continued to be provided there by family and volunteers. Sister Yvonne Ayrey visited the home on a regular basis and assessed Joe, altering the therapy as needed. Joe continued to improve and eventually began to speak, and demonstrated increasing ability in movement, better cognitive function and a great sense of humour.

Fourteen years later, Joe is not back to his pre-accident state, but he can do a great deal, has a wide circle of friends and enjoys life. Was it worth it? Was it worth the time and effort? Did it cost too much? The answers are self-evident.

Joe's parents endured much in addition to the distress directly occasioned by his injuries. Their first challenge came with their fight to avert disconnection of Joe's ventilator. Many other families are overwhelmed by the acute shock of the episode of injury, followed within the week by receipt of a devastating prognosis appended to which is the advice (often given forcefully, as in Joe's case) that the preferred course of 'management' will be to cease life support.

The interval between injury and cessation of support after a preliminary diagnosis that a patient is, and will remain, vegetative varies between intensive care units. Suffice it to observe here that many of the patients in Freeman's files would have fulfilled the criteria for cessation. Using his experience as a guide, there certainly will have been patients similar to Joe among that substantial cohort of people with brain injury from whom support was withdrawn at an early stage on the basis of a very poor prognosis.

The observation that Joe's status seemed to have improved noticeably after the journey to Eastwood serves to direct attention to the environmental deprivation inherent in lying immobilised in a hospital bed. His father's long daily return trip to ensure that Joe received his exercise program from a close family member while at Eastwood was a monumental effort. Freeman has referred on a number of occasions in his writings to the necessity for a family member or friend to adopt the role of a driver who persists as a patient advocate often in the face of contrary medical opinion. Joe's father was an outstanding example of such a driver.

While the procedures in Joe's program were concentrated on regaining physical capacity, the retention of his sense of humour and his comment conveyed to Ted Freeman in a letter from his father that '[l]ife goes on and I wouldn't be dead for quids' indicate that he felt that the prolonged saga had been worthwhile.

Prue's story: Stand up and walk!

Sister Yvonne Ayrey's responsibility at the Brain Injury Therapy Centre at Eastwood was to develop rehabilitation in the patient's home (domiciliary rehabilitation). Yvonne was having outstanding success with her direct, practical and commonsense approach. Yvonne arranged for Prue, who had been in a coma for two months, to come to the Brain Injury Therapy Centre to be assessed. Prue had been in rehabilitation centres and hospitals for two years and 'doctors said nothing more could be done: she would be confined to a wheelchair and need constant institutional care for the rest of her life'. I can recall seeing Prue for the first time. She was sitting in a wheelchair, with her parents, Pat and Ray, standing anxiously beside her. They had been told to place her into a nursing home. Prue was in her early twenties. She was obviously fully aware and understood everything I said to her and, within the limitations of her disability, obeyed all requests. As the assessment was drawing to a close, I looked into Prue's eyes and asked, 'Do you want to go into a nursing home?' She reacted strongly with a look of dismay and slowly she rolled out the words, 'No. I do not want to go into a nursing home!'

I asked Pat and Ray would they be prepared to take their daughter home if we set up a home-based program. They willingly agreed. Tamworth is one of those country towns with a vibrant community and the family was well known in the district, especially since Pat, in her professional capacity, had nursed many of the local people. Within a short time there were 200 volunteers willing to help. They came from all walks of life. Some were professionals, such as nurses, physiotherapists and occupational therapists. Some were farmers and their wives. Some were clerical workers. Some were retired men and women who wanted to help a person in need. They brought with them their delight in watching Prue as she expanded her cognitive and motor abilities. Each one in their turn heartily congratulated this plucky girl as they recognised what she had achieved since their previous visit. After some time, Prue stood up and out of her wheelchair. She slowly learnt to walk with a walking frame and then took a few steps unaided. She helped around the house and took control of her personal care. She resumed work on the computer—which had been her previous occupation. After some time, Prue, who had been a keen horsewoman before her accident, was back in the saddle. Yvonne Ayrey is recorded as saying after Prue had been on a program for one year:

> *She has changed in every aspect. Her balance, her dexterity and her coordination—everything has improved. Her speech is much better and she*

will initiate conversation. She is fit and well and so positive. Prue has a phenomenal driving force that just makes her determined to keep going. She may never be completely like she was before the accident, but she still has years of improvement left and her volunteers seem keen to continue.

While Prue still needs some support, she is now living independently.

Prue's history illustrates the seemingly obvious point that there is nothing to be lost by talking to the patient. On far too many occasions, conversations about a patient deemed to be unaware take place over the patient. As with all the people whose stories are in this group, Prue's rehabilitation occurred at home in familiar surroundings. The description of her volunteer group could most aptly be described as bringing the community to the patient when the patient is unable to go to the community. Another feature of Prue—namely, her 'phenomenal driving force' referred to above—was an essential component of all of these patient stories. In its absence—for instance, in patients whose brain injury is accompanied by clinical depression—the efforts of family and others are unlikely to be as successful as they were in the present group of patients.

Jessie's story: Recovery at home

Jessie was a patient in a major Sydney hospital. A colleague invited me to assess her. She had an unusual type of coma—not from trauma or hypoxia. When I examined her I could find very little evidence of awareness and conveyed this information to my colleague. Jessie came from the country and when it was decided that no more could be done for her she was sent back to the base hospital in the country area, where she remained in the so-called vegetative state. Her husband, Geoff, decided to take her home and set her up on a program there. Yvonne went to show Geoff and the volunteers how to do the program. Slowly, Jessie responded and became more aware. She started to communicate and each time Yvonne went to see her she came back to our weekly meeting highly excited about the changes that were now so positive and so obvious. One day Yvonne was bubbling over and could not contain herself. She said, 'I went to see Jessie. I drove up to her front gate and hopped out of the car. To my amazement, Jessie greeted me at the gate and while clutching my right arm slowly walked with me into her house and sat me down with Geoff. She then made us a cup of tea and produced a cake she had baked to celebrate my coming.'

Jessie continued to improve and I had a letter from Geoff: 'Jessie was the bridesmaid at her sister's wedding. As she walked down the aisle there was not a dry eye in the church. That evening at the reception, Jessie and I waltzed around the floor to a standing ovation.'

Jessie had very little evidence of awareness when examined by Ted Freeman but subsequently regained consciousness after being taken home and then underwent a dramatic recovery. It is not possible to determine whether she may have undergone similar rapid progress in hospital in the absence of a vigorous program of physical and social challenges. From the accounts of other patients, two queries would be legitimate. Would her early signs of awakening have been recognised in a prolonged-care institution? If these had been recognised, to what extent would they have been acted on?

Ian's story: An alternative approach from the start

One night at home we had a phone call from a close friend to say that her son Ian had been riding his bicycle when he was hit by a car and had been admitted to hospital with severe brain injury. Ian's mother, Laurena, came to our home to see us the next day. His father, Bob, was in the United Kingdom on business. The patient was 3 on the Glasgow Coma Scale (the very lowest point). I went into the intensive care ward as a family friend and did manage to carry out a preliminary examination by watching his responses to his mother. Bob returned to Australia as rapidly as possible and, with the help of many friends, the family undertook a modified coma arousal program in the hospital.

The lad remained comatose for six weeks but there were signs that he was arousing. Fifteen weeks after the initial injury he was taken to a rehabilitation hospital where he remained for another six weeks until his parents felt that it would be better for him to be on a home-based program.

When taken home, he was confused and agitated, even aggressive at times. He had markedly decreased awareness and slept for a large part of the day. His facial and emotional expressions were limited and he had difficulty focusing his eyes. He could hold his head upright for only short periods and needed to be strapped into his wheelchair. He was fed through a tube into his stomach and was partially incontinent of bladder and bowels. Sister Yvonne Ayrey set up a program that drew 200 volunteers from friends and neighbours, Knox Grammar School and St John's Presbyterian Church in the Sydney suburb of Wahroonga. My daughter, Susan, helped to nurse him soon after he came home and my wife, Dorothy, became a volunteer.

Slowly, Ian regained his awareness and concentration. He had an enormous drive to get better. The exercises were made user-friendly so that he could accomplish small movements and enjoy that precious sense of achievement. Different exercises were gradually introduced to build on these gains. He commenced to hold his head up for longer periods and sit upright with support in a chair. It was a miraculous day when he stood for the first time. A relearning program was started at his school and he continued to improve in every way. Today, years later, he is married and has full-time employment. It is wonderful to see this brave young man happily making his way in the world.

Ian's parents wrote to the Medical Journal of Australia:[3]

> With this type of injury it must be recognised that the patient's family is also emotionally highly traumatised. In effect there is more than one patient. While traditional patient management systems address the primary patient, the family may be largely left to the dislocation of their life on their own. Being actively involved from the start in the patient's rehabilitation meets the family's need to help their loved one. Incidentally it also makes it easier for them to accept the altered condition of the patient.

> Finally bringing the patient home allows the family to regain a more normal lifestyle. Certainly things are different from the way they were before the accident but the family is making its own changes and is not meeting a routine established by an outside agency—nor is an inordinate amount of time lost in travelling.

Ian's story is one of the most remarkable of the Freeman case histories. His initial neurological status—namely, a score of 3 on the Glasgow Coma Scale—denotes a failure to evince any sign of a response to any of the tests. His prolonged period of unconsciousness compounded this gloomy outlook. Fast forward: years later, he was married and in full-time employment. As emphasised previously, no two patients are identical and, presumably, notwithstanding the ominous features at the outset, the nature of the damage he had sustained, and its extent, left open the possibility of recovery, given adequate opportunities. That these were certainly forthcoming is evident from the description of the program that his parents initiated. Complementing this was the 'enormous drive' referred to in his history.

Conclusion

These patient stories tell of a sequence of events, set in train by the initial episode and which, in the absence of direct intervention, tend to progress, inexorably, to an enduring, dismal outcome. Family intervention, under guidance from Ted Freeman, often interrupted the sequence and enabled a more humane outcome to be achieved.

---

3 Robert Potter & Laurena Potter (1991) Severe brain injury. *Medical Journal of Australia, 153*, 732.

The initial step, following the brain injury that set the sequence in train, was the making of a flawed diagnosis. The nature of that flaw varied between patients. In some instances, the diagnosis of unconsciousness was patently incorrect at the time that it was made. In others, detection of retained, or regained, consciousness required more care, more time and more attention to observations already made by the patient's family members.

The terminology employed in the diagnosis commonly involved the use of the term 'vegetative', a frequent feature in most of the people whom Freeman met throughout his career. Two comments are required in relation to this. The medical literature was not lacking in reports of frequent misdiagnosis of the vegetative state by clinicians with neurological training. To throw around the word 'vegetative' as had been done in referring to many of these patients should have implied that the defined diagnostic guidelines had been observed. Clearly, they were not. The second comment is to stress the ongoing impact that the term could, predictably, be anticipated to have on families.

If categorisation of a person as vegetative failed to depress his or her family, the associated prognosis, generally discounting hopes of recovery, could be relied on to do so. One immediate outcome of this prognosis was likely to be curtailment of acute treatment and sometimes, as in Joe's case, withdrawal of life-support measures.

The gravity of misdiagnosis of any condition will be dependent on factors associated with the inherent difficulty of diagnosing it. Diagnosis of a vegetative state is certainly not simple and the risks of getting it wrong should have inculcated more caution. The ethical opprobrium properly attaching to misdiagnosis, however, derives especially from the completely foreseeable consequences *for patient and family* of the clinician's mistake. The separation, in both time and place, of the acute-care medical setting and the lifetime institutional placement that becomes the fate of poorly assessed patients has ensured that the consequences of misdiagnoses are unlikely to come to the attention of those responsible for making that diagnosis.

A number of patients with brain injury can remain fully conscious, albeit unable to communicate, and are considered to be 'locked in' as a direct effect of the original injury. Another group of patients can be locked in by the healthcare system. Aggravation of the patient's original disability by commitments to minimal care during the acute-care phase can effectively result in 'locking in' of people who have the capacity for a much fuller life. The example of Cecil's case, given above, illustrates how initial failure to treat fractures, because of diagnostic inadequacy, curtailed his chances of a considerably improved lifestyle in later years.

The possible outcomes of long-term treatment designed to provide stimulation and to encourage a person to regain skills that will facilitate increased independence were well shown in a number of the patients discussed above. Others in this group probably had similar potential, but circumstances curtailed its realisation. As noted above by Ted Freeman, not all of the people whom he was asked to meet appeared to have any detectable consciousness and, accordingly, were not entered into programs.

Finally, as an indication of what might be possible, the remarkable story of the patient Ian deserves attention. Given the variety of brain injuries which, while clinically similar, can entail differing degrees of damage, it is not legitimate to use a case history of one conventionally managed patient as a control for assessing the value of a Freeman program for another patient. Nevertheless, Ian's abysmal score on the Glasgow Coma Scale contrasts strikingly with his excellent outcome, and points to the possibilities that may be opened up by very early initiation of a program. This is not often permissible when a patient is in an intensive care unit. If some degree of stimulation is feasible at this early stage without interfering with a patient's treatment, there could be a good case for undertaking it. The letter from Ian's parents in the *Medical Journal of Australia* makes the case well.

3. Families: No easy way forward

Any reading of the preceding chapter is likely to leave a strong impression that the families of the patients whose stories are summarised were very much part of those stories. The frequently cited adage that a severe brain injury inevitably affects more than one life springs out of the pages. Family responses can range from utter despair and literally walking away from the affected member consigned to a nursing home or similar institution to a total commitment to attempts to rehabilitate him or her, usually at home.

It does not require too much reflection to realise that there are major impacts on a patient's family. First-order consequences are likely to be psychological and economic. Second-order consequences may involve intra-family relations, educational and career aspirations of a patient's siblings and changes in the lifestyle patterns and employment opportunities of all members. The precise nature of the consequences is likely to depend on the relationship of the patient to other family members.

This chapter is based on a collection of letters written by family members. The patient stories in the preceding chapter were reproduced unedited from Ted Freeman's account and incorporate the insights and experience gained from working with a large group of patients with brain injuries. In contrast, the stories that follow provide an account of a young person's progress after brain injury as perceived by the family for whom all of this represented a new experience. These family accounts have been drawn from a collection of letters written in 1995 and addressed to a federal parliamentarian who had expressed interest in learning about Freeman's approach to assisting people with brain injuries.

A total of 53 such letters were examined when selecting those presented below. Applying a selection process to such material may be criticised on the basis that it has been slanted to favour particular points of view. If one were purporting to draw statistically valid conclusions, this criticism would be justified; however, the intent of this selection is to present a qualitative description of the wide variety of impacts, positive and negative, of patient–family interactions.

Of the collection of letters, 35 came from one or both parents; 12 were written by a spouse. Three came from volunteers who had participated in programs, two from siblings and one from the patient himself. He is a remarkable young man with great IT skills. The age profile of the patients was almost completely in the first three decades of life, with the youngest aged three. The circumstances of the brain injury were overwhelmingly motor vehicle accidents (around 80 per cent), with smaller numbers attributable to strokes, physical assaults, cardiac arrest, asphyxia and epileptic seizures.

Additional information, concerning the impressions of families who had participated in Freeman's programs, details a group of responses from patients' families to a short questionnaire circulated by Ted Freeman. Once again, no claims of statistical validity are made but the tabulated responses record lived experiences. Finally, a letter outlining one family's conclusions, composed by the parents of Joe, whose story was presented in the previous chapter, is a realistic account of experiences many of which were certainly shared by others. Attention is also directed to the published letter from Ian's parents, which was reproduced in the previous chapter.

To anticipate the thrust of the letters and recapitulate the nature of the consequences described in the preceding chapter, it is apparent that the sudden occurrence of a life-threatening brain injury will have a major, frequently devastating, psychological impact on other members of a family. When the affected person remains unconscious for a prolonged period, this impact will be aggravated. The receipt of a prognosis that is, at best, extremely guarded and commonly dismissive of any hope of recovery will augment this reaction. At this time, family responses may split in different directions. Some people commit to trying everything possible to assist the family member; others accept medical advice, often given within weeks of the accident, to commit a patient to a nursing home, institution for the terminally ill or similar and then to 'walk away and forget'. Others waver between positions.

Some of the most trenchant criticism of Freeman, examined below, has been that his approach engenders 'false hope' in the first group of families. Implicit in this argument is the notion that false hope will worsen the major psychological impacts on a family. A more balanced consideration of consequences for a family must acknowledge that psychological impacts on those electing to 'walk away and forget' may be at least as significant and quite possibly more depressing. Walking away may be easy; forgetting may not be.

It does not require a doctorate in psychology to anticipate that repressed and unresolved grieving among those who accept the advice to abandon a relative may well outlast the disappointment in the 'Freeman group' if there is no success after they give it their best shot. I am not aware of any published long-term follow-up interviews with the 'walk away' group. It would certainly require extraordinary sensitivity and considerable resources to undertake such research.

The predictable economic consequences for a family of caring for a member with acquired brain injury will vary with the position of the patient in the family.

When the patient is the breadwinner, the immediate effects of loss of income will be obvious. Comparable impacts may occur if the breadwinner decides to forgo paid employment in order to play a lead role in family members' attempts to rehabilitate the patient. Insurance payouts to cover care of the patient are not always available at an early stage if there are disputes about liability. Some patients have not been eligible for compensation at any time.

If the parents of a patient who has sustained a severe brain injury devote a large part of their time to implementing a rehabilitation program, the patient's siblings may feel deprived of parental attention. Straitened family financial circumstances may threaten siblings' educational aspirations. In some instances, a severe brain injury may strengthen family cohesion but in others it may become a disruptive influence. All of these consequences for a family undertaking a domiciliary rehabilitation program crop up in the family letters but attention in selecting the extracts has been concentrated on the tenacity exhibited in their concern and care for the injured member.

Brian's story

Whilst some families opted to take their patient home because of dissatisfaction with institutional rehabilitation, Brian's parents were forced to do so when funding of his care was ceased abruptly. In the event, the experience he had at home subsequently could not have been provided within an institutional environment.

Brian was seventeen when he was critically injured in a motor vehicle accident, two years before this letter was written. Describing his course in an intensive care unit, his parents recalled:

> He had numerous operations and we were told by medical staff that he was 'brain dead' and had a 3% chance of survival. After six weeks, our son remained in a deep coma with a prognosis of severe brain damage. The doctors told us that they were to hold an executive meeting to decide whether to turn off Brian's life support. We were horrified. Three days after this meeting the neurologist said his chances of survival had increased to 10%.

> In desperation we contacted Dr Ted Freeman ... [he] assessed Brian and we commenced a coma arousal programme with some 35 volunteers.

Brian was transferred to the rehabilitation section of another hospital where he remained for 12 months.

> We continued to carry out Dr Freeman's coma arousal therapy program
> with Dr Freeman visiting Brian fortnightly and changing the program
> on a regular basis as Brian improved.

At this time the insurance company funding Brian's hospital costs indicated that
it would no longer do so. Faced with a choice of bringing him home or placing
him in a nursing home, his parents opted for the former.

> We were told by the rehabilitation doctor that Brian would never have
> any quality of life, particularly that he would never have his traciostomy
> [sic] tube removed. He would never eat orally and would always have
> to be fed through a gastrostomy tube. The trachiostomy [sic] tube
> was removed under instruction of the Ear, Nose and Throat Specialist
> approximately three weeks before Brian left hospital. Since Brian has
> been at home we have been able to slowly introduce solid foods orally
> and he now eats normal family meals. Although Brian cannot speak he is
> very alert and aware of what is going on. He expresses happiness, anger,
> frustration, sadness, anxiety and is just learning to communicate yes
> and no with basic head nods. He enjoys watching his surfing videos, Mr
> Bean and several TV shows.

> Our volunteers now number approximately 50 and they carry out
> two therapy sessions daily devised by Dr Freeman. The first session is
> usually carried out by ladies and involves fine motor skills, identifying
> colours, words and photos, doing puzzles etc. The second session is
> very physical and usually carried out by Brian's school friends and
> other men. It involves Brian standing unaided, rolling him over a barrel,
> peddling an exercise bike and helping Brian to regain his balance. Brian
> also has daily physiotherapy, weekly martial arts, weekly massage and
> fortnightly speech pathology.

> Although no one can accurately predict Brian's future capabilities he has
> certainly come a long way and exceeded all expectations.

A first comment on the program in which Brian has been entered could relate
to its intensity. It would be among the best in this respect, but this assessment
should be immediately qualified by noting that there are many among the best
in the letters. A second observation could address the vigorous nature of the
sessions carried out by Brian's school friends. While feasible for a nineteen-year-
old patient with a previous history of considerable physical activity, it would
probably be impractical for a 'typical' forty-year-old. Against this, attention
could be drawn to the preponderance of younger people (that is, under thirty)
among patients affected by severe brain injury after motor vehicle accidents

and then entered into programs recommended by Freeman. Coincidentally, it follows that this cohort of young patients will have the most to endure, in terms of duration, if committed to a nursing home.

Reading his parents' account of Brian's emotions and daily activities some two years after his accident, questions may be raised about his quality of life. If so, it would be appropriate to recall the remark of Dr Keith Andrews of the Royal Hospital for Neurodisability in London to the effect that if one of his patients had a view of his own quality of life that differed from his (that is, Andrews') then he (Andrews) must be wrong. A closing observation on the account given by Brian's parents would relate to the utter improbability that such a labour-intensive rehabilitation would ever be practicable within the formal healthcare system.

Inevitably, this raises a question of resource allocation—namely, whether some diversion of support from a medical goal of 'curing' into slow-stream non-institutional 'caring' rehabilitation targeted towards achieving the best possible quality of life should occur when an individual's prognosis is pessimistic.

Dallas's story

Dallas's story provides a striking example of the feasibility of achieving a worthwhile improvement in a person's life experience notwithstanding long delay in instituting a domiciliary rehabilitation program. It also emphasises that a family may consider that the stresses associated with long-term, intensive support in the home may be more acceptable than the ongoing stress following permanent placement in a nursing home.

Dallas sustained severe brain injuries in a motor vehicle accident at the age of sixteen. This was seven years before his parents contacted Freeman. Their comment on the first meeting was 'no promise of rainbows but good strong advice'. Before this meeting, they 'became desperate to find help for Dallas who had been written off by medical staff from the very beginning'. Following the first meeting:

> We began the program in 1992 with good solid hard work with 60 volunteers. Now [1995] we are at the stage where Dallas has dropped the program because he can attend a fitness gym and work with a trainer. Recently Dallas had his legs lengthened by having his knees straightened because the tendons had shortened due to sitting so long [seven years] in a wheelchair.

Dallas's mother provided her analysis of the program: 'You may wonder what this program is. Well I, Dallas and our helpers liken it to good hard physical training and social contact that these isolated people get after sitting around for years doing nothing.'

This analysis is close to that quoted above from Brian's parents. Dallas's mother reflected that:

> Some people say this type of program is very hard on the family but what we say is not being able to get help is terrible and seeing the patient lying around and knowing that they could do more if only the help was available.

The stress that such programs place on families like those of Dallas and Brian must be considered in the light of the psychological stress, alluded to above, which could well be the lot of families who have taken the advice to 'walk away and forget'. A concluding observation from Dallas's mother on his behalf has much wider applicability:

> From the time that Dallas had his accident he was treated as a cereble [sic] palsy child, instead of as a recovering accident victim. Someone even said recently to our daughter 'Oh he should be with a psychiatrist as all head injured people are'. I ask you how will we ever be able to educate people that not all head injured people are the same.

This is a profound insight from a patient's mother.

John's story

John was removed from the 'conventional' rehabilitation system because of his parents' dissatisfaction with it. While he remained severely limited, he was able to resume life as a member of a family, something that was of great value to his parents and to John.

John was involved in a motor vehicle accident at the age of twelve. His father recalled:

> The advice—he would be at best vegetative and it would be best to place him in a nursing home [at the age of twelve]. He stayed in hospital for six months. It was a difficult period for my wife and myself, both emotionally and physically. We had the trauma of trying to accept his condition and the final outcome, the financial concerns for ongoing care [the circumstances of John's accident were such that third-party insurance was not prepared to accept liability, and medical insurance,

believing it to be an insurance case, would not meet costs] and the long hours of hospital visits and still maintaining a semblance of normal family life for two other children at home.

After John spent six months in an acute-care hospital, his parents succeeded in having him accepted into what was described to them as the 'most switched on rehab. centre for head injuries' (in Sydney in the early 1980s). John's father wrote:

> Oh how depressing it was for him to spend the next four months propped up with pillows! My wife could not tolerate the inactivity and used to spend six hours a day with him giving him passive exercise. She was reminded by the authorities that 'she wasn't covered by worker's compensation'. Furthermore she was counselled that she was an over anxious and over expectant mother. At ten months John began to respond to command[s] and made meaningful movements and commenced to communicate.

Two points require comment. John's mother was undertaking passive exercises with him for prolonged periods each day. This could be read as an activity similar to those undertaken by many other parents in the course of a program suggested by Ted Freeman, except for one detail. This occurred some two years before the family established contact with Freeman. To explain this independently evolved similarity some decades later, my suggestion is that both practices—Freeman's programs and John's mother's interventions—were initiated in response to an intuitive belief that they could possibly help the patient. This belief may have been initiated by incidental observations of improvement that were reinforced subsequently by their persistence and gradual augmentation as a program continued.

Some two years after their experience in the 'switched on' rehabilitation centre, John's parents made contact with Freeman:

> With Ted we felt for the first time that someone understood our situation and was prepared to offer a programme of rehabilitation for our son. John attended the Brain Injury Therapy Centre in Eastwood for over three years and steadily made progress which improved his quality of life and allowed us to successfully care for him in the home environment. It was with disappointment that we saw the Centre close for lack of funding. In our case we carried on with a home program with community volunteers and following the rehabilitation therapy learned at the Centre. Ted Freeman continued to visit at home and advise.

John's father has succinctly indicated the gains he associated with his son's time at the Brain Injury Therapy Centre. This was considerably less than enabling

John to establish an independent lifestyle, but was nevertheless considered to be valuable—it became feasible to care for him in the home environment. Whilst some commentators might dismiss this as an inadequate return for the parents' effort, John's parents did not. The closing assessment from John's father was emphatic: 'Today at the age of twenty five, John while still severely incapacitated, still follows a daily home programme, still improves a little, keeps healthy, enjoys life and is a happy soul.'

John's story draws attention to the value a family can attach to a limited recovery sufficient to permit a young person to resume life as a member following a severe brain injury. Many brain injured people who participate in intensive rehabilitation programs may be in this category.

Matthew's story

Matthew's story provides an example of the value of what, in some medical assessments, might be considered a very limited recovery. The value of that recovery for his family was enhanced by its occurrence after a very discouraging beginning.

After sustaining a brain injury in a motor vehicle accident at the age of ten, Matthew remained in coma for three months. His parents recalled their early experience: 'After speaking to the hospital doctors, we were advised to forget our son and walk away because he wouldn't improve. We were also advised that rehabilitation hospitals would not accept him because he was too bad.'

Matthew's family contacted Freeman and brought their son home, where they undertook a rehabilitation program. Seven years after his accident, Matthew's mother wrote:

> Our son is still in a wheelchair but gives us love and laughter and is still improving. He goes out on social outings. He also goes to craft lessons. It's been a very hard seven years for our family, also for our son, but the hard work has shown success. If we had listened to the hospital doctors, our son would still have been in a nursing home, locked away from the outside world at the age of 17 years.

It would require a fairly two-dimensional mind-set to attempt to quantify Matthew's quality of life, which is essentially a judgment to be made by the subject and the family. Such an assessment will be likely to consider the individual within the family. 'Conventional' medical assessment will never be able to assess the value of the lives of people such as John and Matthew because this would necessarily entail insight into mutual interactions between the individual and other family members. The impact of the presence of the injured person on relationships between other family members would also be very relevant.

Leah's story

This story exemplifies the way in which a family's distress following accidental injury to a daughter can be compounded by a premature negative prognosis; however, it also illustrates the way in which refusal by a family to accept that prognosis, accompanied by retention of hope, led to dogged persistence, with attempts to help her.

Leah was involved in a motor vehicle accident at the age of nineteen. She suffered multiple injuries and the extent of her brain injury was not apparent for a week. In retrospect, her father considered that this delayed recognition had averted pressure to make decisions about the continuation of life support. The extent of her brain injury became apparent when her sedation was withdrawn and she did not wake up. Leah's father recalled:

> The doctors felt then that she had suffered lack of oxygen at the scene of the accident and there was no way to assess the extent of this damage. So started our grief, anxiety and uncertainty with little encouragement about any way to help Leah. Her mother refused to listen to the doctors that nothing would be done until Leah woke up. She felt in her heart that there must be a way to wake her daughter.

> Then out of the blue a friend told us about Dr Freeman and lent his copy of Dr Freeman's book to us. We were able to understand Leah's problem and found great relief in realising there may be a way to help Leah. When approaching Leah's doctors I was surprised to find them cold to the idea of another doctor assessing Leah. I finally got permission for Dr Freeman to see her. This turned sour on the day he arrived as the head of the hospital department refused to let him assess Leah, despite her doctor's reluctant permission. Luckily Dr Freeman was able to assess Leah if he promised not to touch her.

> After his assessment we were given a program to help stimulate Leah's senses. To us this was the first positive action in helping Leah. I must say that despite disapproval we were allowed to implement these exercises. Family and friends worked together in trying to get a response from Leah. After many weeks of loving care Leah started to respond. Dr Freeman kept the exercises up to date and Leah finally awoke, but still there was very little recognition from Leah.

We kept the exercises up day and night. We never left Leah without trying to get a response. More heartbreak came when we were told Leah would only have two choices after leaving the hospital, a nursing home or constant care at our home. We kept up the program knowing that many of the hospital staff felt it was hopeless.

Leah's response was sufficiently promising that it was decided she could be sent to a rehabilitation centre in another city rather than to a nursing home. After two months, it was felt that Leah was missing her parents' daily presence and that, consequently, it would be better for her to return home. At the time of writing his letter, her father summarised her status as follows:

Leah is now able to dress herself, toilet herself and three weeks ago she took her first steps on her own. It is still hard to understand her when she talks, but when she says: 'Dad, Mum, I love you more than you ever will know'. I break down and weep inside.

As with any individual patient, it is impossible to declare with certainty that this attention *caused* her gradual awakening. What *can* be said with considerable confidence is that *recognition* of the first signs, and hence the resultant intensive efforts of family and friends to encourage the progress of her returning awareness and responsiveness to others, would have been much less likely, if not improbable, in the absence of those efforts.

Leah's father's account of her emotional response to her parents, given its dependence on higher brain function, testifies to the quality of her mental recovery. The sense of achievement of both patient and parents with what some might consider to be relatively modest results emphasises again the issue of *who* is entitled to judge progress.

Paul's story

Paul's family, like all of those whose story is recounted in this chapter, was confronted with a choice of 'nursing home or take him home'. The latter course, which they adopted, imposed great day-to-day difficulties on them, but their persistence was reinforced by their reflections on the likely nature of his existence as a young man in a nursing home.

Paul sustained brain injuries in a motor vehicle accident when aged twenty-one. Four years later, his parents recalled the assessment of his doctors at the time:

While we can never really tell, Paul has suffered a very severe brain injury and the chances of his recovery to any significant degree would appear remote. Paul could neither move nor communicate at this time and his breathing pattern was still erratic and of concern.

His early course was problematic: 'His progress was limited and twice he was returned to the intensive care unit following breathing difficulties.'

After four weeks, Paul's suitability for rehabilitation was assessed as 'borderline' but he was transferred to a rehabilitation centre. His response was erratic. Some 10 months after Paul's admission, his parents were told that Paul's improvement to that time suggested that he was unlikely to benefit from further rehabilitation and, consequently, he was to be discharged. The advice at that time was: 'Place Paul in a nursing home or take him home and care for him, but we wouldn't recommend that as his improvement will be negligible and it will be emotionally intolerable for you as parents.'

At this time Paul's parents heard of Ted Freeman and contacted him:

> With much apprehension but with Ted's guidance and support we elected to care for Paul at our home. Ted had suggested that the home environment would automatically provide a positive catalyst toward Paul's wellbeing and this was evident at a very early stage.

Caring for Paul at home necessitated his mother giving up paid employment and his father taking on part-time employment, and this, together with the lack of compensation, severely constrained family finances. His parents wrote:

> Ted's long experience in the area of brain injury enabled him to introduce practical, effective strategies, not always based on traditional medical assumptions, which converted to what we now call 'a voluntary home based rehabilitation program'. This involved sourcing volunteers, dedicating part of our home to Paul's activities and rostering helpers around Paul's variable and unpredictable attitudes. With enormous assistance from our volunteers, who numbered over 100 at one stage, we initiated a re-training program for Paul as well as providing the 24 hour care he required for his personal inadequacies (bed and clothing changes 3 times each night were not uncommon in the early stages). The results some two and a half years after the program was initiated have been worth it as Paul can now walk with assistance, feed himself, play a variety of computer games, go out (accompanied) to restaurants and movies and he is no longer required to take medication. While he still can not speak he can utter phrases and is totally aware of what goes on around him.

They reflected: 'What would have been his lot in a nursing home at 21 years of age?'

Paul's progress during an extended period in a rehabilitation centre did not produce sufficient improvement to justify its continuation. The account of his program at home should dispel any notions that domiciliary rehabilitation will be a simple matter. The dedication shown by Paul's family was extraordinary, although not exceptional. The closing reflection from their letter concerning his fate if in a nursing home is sobering.

Christine's story

In common with the preceding stories, Christine's involved initial discouragement followed by family assumption of the rehabilitation role. What her story does document especially well is the enhancement of lifestyle that she achieved. One senses that her parents' comparisons of her swimming and riding prowess were not with what she could undertake before her accident but with her enormous limitations when discharged from hospital.

Christine was involved in a motor vehicle accident at the age of sixteen and remained unconscious for six weeks. Her father's letter contained many of the features already noted from the preceding five family letters, for example: 'Doctors told us that she would be a "vegetable" for the rest of her life and would never get out of bed so book her into a nursing home and get on with your lives.'

On Christine's discharge from hospital, a Freeman-planned home rehabilitation program with a team of volunteers was organised and, nine years after the accident, Christine was described as 'leading a happy lifestyle', which included walking, talking, swimming and riding (bicycle and horse). Two comments in her father's letter are quite thought provoking:

> The argument has been put forward that Dr Freeman's methods have not been scientifically proven. One of the main reasons would seem to be a 'control' element in his experiments. Well all I can say is that there are vast numbers of patients which have been given very little if any treatment by the brain injury specialists which are admirably suited to be considered as 'control'.

This is surely a small dose of commonsense from a non-medical commentator with personal experience of brain injury.

The father's letter concluded with a recollection from a Brain Injury Council of Australia conference held in Canberra several years previously:

The chair of the session asked 'Is there anyone present who has sustained brain injury who would like to address this conference?' A man stood with difficulty from his wheelchair and said 'I would like to say to the medical profession—you have done a wonderful job in saving my life—but for God's sake help me do something with my life!'

Common features in parents' letters

The letters that provided these extracts are typical of those of the 53 respondents. Several features are common. A diagnosis as 'vegetative' seems to have been freely given. As mentioned in Chapter 2, the adoption of this description in non-medical conversation may be feeding back into medical practice and resulting often in its loose use. Of overwhelming importance from the family's perspective is the highly emotive connotation attached to the term vegetative. This was inadequately considered, I believe, by those who pioneered the term but, given that it has become entrenched in medical jargon, anyone using it when talking with a family should be aware of its emotional impact and handle the consultation process very carefully. In practice, this appears not to have occurred in many instances.

The outlook for many of the patients represented in this and the preceding chapter was certainly not good when families were briefed by medical personnel. It would be unreasonable to expect those personnel to dissemble on this point. Few, if any, of the doctors responsible for early management, be they intensivists or neurosurgeons, would ever have had the opportunity of meeting a single one of the patients described in these two chapters, or the considerably larger group whom they represent, some years after they sustained an injury. Consequently, it is not to be expected that they could indicate that, notwithstanding the gloomy prognosis that they were then providing, they had had personal experience of one patient who had actually regained a standard of life which that patient and family considered to be worth having, despite having been accorded a similarly gloomy prognosis. This recollection would probably be accompanied by the caveat that such an outcome represented a very long shot. Whilst imprecise use of the 'v' word is regrettable, the advice to the parents of a twelve-year-old child to find a nursing home placement can only be categorised as closed minded, since alternative evidence was available. It would also imply considerable insensitivity on the part of the medical practitioner at the time of discussing prognosis with a patient's family. Ted Freeman has drawn attention to a compelling description of this predicament in the following terms:

The US National Head Injury Foundation Newsletter *provides a picture of the quandary of the family when thrown precipitately into brain injury:*

It is impossible to remain aloof when faced with a family, torn by fright and anger, handicapped by guilt and denial and seemingly abandoned by a system which does not care enough.

All seven of the patients whose family letters were discussed above were alive at the time when those letters were written. A person who has sustained a brain injury of the severity that occasioned a family approach to Freeman may die suddenly and unexpectedly, for example, with respiratory failure as a delayed consequence of brain-stem injury, after years of gradual recovery.

The vicissitudes encountered during attempts to set up a clinical trial of the efficacy of Ted Freeman's approach to helping people with severe brain injuries are outlined in Chapter 6. When a number of families were undertaking domiciliary rehabilitation programs under his supervision, Freeman developed a questionnaire to seek information from them about their impressions of their program. He summarised the results of a simple questionnaire:

Medicine, like most professions, is greatly influenced by statistics. It is only when numbers are available that professionals appear to be able to meet and discuss matters in common. I decided to prepare a questionnaire for 38 families currently receiving therapy at home and I based it on the questionnaire devised by Macquarie University for its Coma Care Family survey. It would have been preferable for my survey to come from an independent source, but I could not get any authorities interested.

I asked the families:

Question 1. Before you started the program were you told by the doctors that the patient was, or would be, vegetative? The replies, all of which were provided by families, were:

Almost always or usually: 33 (87 per cent)

Seldom: 0 (0 per cent)

Never: 5 (13 per cent)

Of the 33 who had replied almost always or usually:

- *29 of the 33 patients now obeyed commands*
- *26 of the 33 patients now could speak*
- *23 of the 33 patients now could weight transfer (take some weight on their legs)*
- *13 of the 33 patients now were walking*
- *22 of the 33 patients now could feed themselves.*

Question 2. Before you started the program were you told by the doctors that the patient would be in a nursing home for the rest of their life? The replies were:

Almost always or usually: 35 (92 per cent)

Seldom: 1 (3 per cent)

Never: 2 (5 per cent)

In fact, 29 of these 35 (77 per cent) patients were now at home.

There was a marked demarcation between those who answered almost always or usually in contrast with those who answered seldom or never. The result was very clear-cut.

I knew that this survey did not prove anything scientifically, but it seemed to justify a more aggressive and positive approach to those people with severe brain injury. I showed the results to several medical colleagues. They remained unimpressed. They pointed out that because I had done the research, it was suspect. They also said I had selected the patients to be assessed. I thought this to be a non-argument. They repeated to me that they considered a double-blind controlled prospective study was the only acceptable research. I felt enormously frustrated at such limited thinking. It appeared totally unethical and immoral for the medical profession to allow a continuing stream of severely brain injured patients to be consigned to nursing homes while they waited for years to produce a foolproof research document. I fumed, but had to bite my tongue. There was nothing else I could do.

Freeman's colleagues had a point but, paradoxically, when their criticism is followed through the only interpretation that can be placed on it runs directly counter to that which they intended. Of course, this is a selected group of patients. They were, effectively, twice selected. In the first instance, they were *selected out* by the medical gatekeepers of the Australian healthcare system. As already explained, the seven family letters, extracts from which were cited above, were selected from a file of 53. These seven were not selected because they were a minority presenting Freeman and his practices in the most favourable light. Rather, they are representative of the whole group of letters. Moreover, the chosen seven best lent themselves to a relatively succinct citation appropriate for a book. The message conveyed starkly in every letter in the file is that the family was told to make arrangements for long-term care without hope of recovery.

The respondents in Freeman's group of 38 families were selected a second time. This second selection process entailed *their selection* of Freeman as a medical practitioner who, perhaps, had something to offer. This selection process was categorically not influenced by Freeman. Whilst it is now more acceptable for medical professionals to display their wares with the assistance of the advertising industry, Freeman's philosophy and practices were not disseminated in the media. He certainly lacked the resources to do so; I suspect that this practice was, in any case, contrary to principles that he and his contemporaries absorbed in medical school. The families who sought his help had not been referred by medical practitioners. On the contrary, some had been actively discouraged from doing so by their doctors.

Questions of selection bias aside, the responses provided by families to Freeman's questionnaire bear strong resemblance to those much fuller descriptions that have been extracted above from family letters.

The case history notes of the patient Joe from Ted Freeman's records (Chapter 2) are supplemented with a record of the saga for his parents in the form of a series of notes compiled by his father and sent to Freeman.

The notes show as follows.

1. Our fight with the doctors to keep Joe on life support for a little longer.

2. Our fight with the doctors and staff at … hospital to keep treating Joe. They were just going to let him die.

3. Our first meeting with you gave us some hope but we had to overcome problems to get you in to see Joe.

4. We had problems getting a shunt fitted. It was fitted only after we demanded that you see Joe.

5. After spending a day at Eastwood we decided it was what Joe needed as he had made no progress in the public system.

6. When we first saw Joe at Eastwood, I recall you put a comb in Joe's hand and after some prompting you asked Joe what he did with the comb. He started to comb his hair. This was the first positive move Joe had made. This brought tears to my eyes as I realised Joe did have some hope.

7. From that point on Joe made good progress under your guidance and after five months came home to a home program.

8. Joe continued to improve and we made a move to Queensland where Joe soon became a very respected member of the town being an employer, a substantial rate payer and a taxpayer [Joe's parents had used some of his compensation money to buy him a small farm].

9. At this point in time Joe's fund was controlled by the NSW Public Trustee who we found unsatisfactory. After six and a half years the fund was transferred to [the] Queensland Public Trustee where we are now looking at rebuilding the fund to what it was before.

10. Joe's life is a happy one even though he is confined to a wheelchair and he often says, 'Life goes on and I wouldn't be dead for quids.'

In his assessment of life, Joe was at one with Keith Andrews, Director of the Royal Hospital for Neurodisability at Putney, UK. In the course of an interview with a reporter, Andrews remarked: 'Quality of life is something I have, not something you tell me I have.'[1]

Conclusion

The accounts given above by families who have lived with a member who has survived a severe brain injury with substantial disabilities offer insights into this experience that statistics cannot capture. The almost invariably banal negativity of the prognostication in the early stages was often followed, at a later stage, by exclusion from rehabilitation systems that lacked adaptability to the needs and potential of the individual. The requirement for patients to conform to a system that prioritised 'cure' over 'care' often reflected a closing of the bureaucratic mind.

Criticism of Freeman's approach to rehabilitation of people, such as those whose stories have been recalled in this and the preceding chapter, has often directed considerable attention to the welfare of patients' families. Interviewing of families by competent professionals, which will be discussed in a later chapter, has found that the initial event of the accident responsible for brain injury has commonly been the most traumatic event in a family's experience.

One criticism of Freeman's approach has been that it may engender 'false hope' in participating families. At least three responses to this proposition appear to be appropriate. First, as exemplified above, many of the people for whom domiciliary programs were undertaken achieved outcomes which they, and their families, regarded as worthwhile.

---

1   Jeremy Laurance (1996) Vegetative state diagnosis wrong in many patients. *The Times* [London], 5 July.

A second response, applicable to families who committed to programs that did not produce significant improvement, concerns the nature of hope. I believe that a strong case exists for the value of hope, even when this is not ultimately realised. It is too simplistic to assert that the only value of hope is determined by its ultimate outcome. Hope is a possession that can afford support throughout the period of its currency, irrespective of whether the aspirations underlying it are ultimately achieved. The benefits accruing during that period are unlikely to be retrospectively ablated if the hoped-for outcome does not eventuate. One benefit may be a gradual adjustment to its non-achievement. It is appropriate to recall an earlier evaluation:

> Hope is itself a species of happiness, perhaps the chief happiness which this world affords: but, like all other pleasures immoderately enjoyed, the excesses of hope must be expiated by pain; and expectations improperly indulged, must end in disappointment.[2]

A third response to the 'false hope' contention, which has featured in the literature on the subject, is to direct attention to the psychological impact of a decision to abandon the affected family member to an inappropriate placement for the duration of his or her life. I find it difficult to dismiss the probability that, if there has previously been close intra-family bonding, other family members are likely to remain subject to recurrent episodes of remorse. In contrast, families who have hoped and tried unsuccessfully to bring those hopes to fruition can resume life with the reassurance that they have done their best. From some personal observation, I suspect that families who have lost a member after a concerted mutual effort are ultimately at peace in a way that others who followed the 'walk away' advice never can be.

An issue that will inevitably be raised by stories similar to those touched on in this chapter is that of the value to be attached to the lives of patients who remain considerably disabled after a domiciliary program. In evaluating the value of the life of such a person, I believe that one should take account of the quality of his or her life, of the experience of that family and, most importantly, of the quality of the *interaction* between patient and family during the time which they shared. Any aggregation of the life expectancy in years of people with severe brain injuries cannot capture the value of those years in which the family walked the path together, often experiencing a variety of hardships.

A general question raised by family stories is that of resource allocation. Domiciliary rehabilitation, as undertaken by families following a 'Freeman program', requires a commitment in carer hours, which, if undertaken on a paid basis, would be far beyond the scope of any health budget. It is, nevertheless,

---

2   Samuel Johnson (1953) Letter to a lady soliciting patronage, 8/6/1762, in *Boswell's Life of Johnson* Oxford University Press, Oxford, 261.

quite likely that the value of the work entailed by domiciliary care and rehabilitation will elude economic measurement in much the same way as occurs with housework. Furthermore, the environment of a healthcare institution could not provide the reassurance and security to a severely incapacitated person that is provided by a familiar home environment.

If the role of the healthcare system is envisaged primarily as that of achieving cures within a certain time, perhaps it is reasonable to redirect some budgetary support to assisting slow-stream rehabilitation located outside hospitals and institutions designed to provide aged care. The potential, described in the family stories above, to recruit volunteers to implement this could result in significant lessening of the financial burden on the healthcare system. Ideally, one might envisage a carefully planned transition from hospital to a more appropriate setting as an accredited pathway for people whose possible rehabilitation was expected to be prolonged.

4. Emergence from coma after brain injury: Freeman's contribution

This chapter discusses the initial events during emergence from coma and the ongoing strategies that Freeman adopted to facilitate this. In each case, it is intended to recount the story of his contribution to the advancement of recovery at these two stages of the process, whenever possible, using his own words.

As a background, the beliefs and practices inherent in managing comatose patients in the early 1980s are touched on. The inferences drawn by Freeman, acting on the basis of observation, to shorten the duration of coma, are examined in the light of studies employing brain scanning to study consciousness, a quarter-century later. In more than one instance, his empiricism will be seen to have been remarkably prescient.

Imposing a distinction between initial emergence from coma when a person is recovering from brain injury and subsequent improvements in the level of awareness and ability to engage in everyday activities may be biologically artificial. The distinction, however, is useful, even though emergence and subsequent improvement could essentially be parts of a continuum, as the differing management considerations, traditionally prevailing, justify their consideration in separate chapters.

Whilst Australian mainstream teaching and practice in the 1980s held that early intervention with the intention of expediting the emergence of patients with brain injury from coma was pointless, the medical literature was not lacking in suggestions that there could be advantages in alternative approaches. A 1968 review by Carl Carlsson and colleagues in the *Journal of Neurosurgery* identified a consistent association between the length of time during which a person remained in coma and the eventual level of recovery.[1]

It has not been possible to apportion causation when attempting to interpret this association. Furthermore, the nature of the observed association was not necessarily similar in all the cases reviewed by Carlsson et al. According to one interpretation, the duration of coma may be entirely a reflection of the severity of the initial traumatic damage. An alternative interpretation is that prolongation of coma might aggravate the initial damage. If this second explanation gains acceptance as applicable in some cases, interventions intended to shorten the period of coma can be considered.

---

1   Carl Carlsson, Claes von Essen & Jan Lofgren (1968) Factors affecting the clinical course of patients with severe head injuries. *Journal of Neurosurgery, 29*, 242.

Ideally, it would be preferable to identify in advance those cases in which intervention would be worthwhile. On the other hand, if there is nothing to suggest that intervention might introduce risks to any patient, identification of those who are most likely to benefit becomes less important; however, it might be argued that, notwithstanding the minimal likelihood of risk to the individual subject from early intervention, its general application might incur a waste of limited health system resources.

On the assumption that little can be achieved in the process of rehabilitation until a patient has emerged from coma, a distinction has commonly been drawn between measures appropriate in the management of a comatose patient and those to be adopted after emergence is first observed. For instance, Jacquelin Perry differentiated between measures to be adopted whilst a patient remains in coma and unresponsive, and those which might profitably be instituted at a later stage. Referring to the first stage, she advised that '[p]reventive rehabilitation is designed to minimise the complications of inactivity that tend to develop during a protracted curative process (contractures, pressure sores, muscle atrophy, cardiopulmonary deconditioning, cognitive dulling)'.[2] She recommended that when the patient became responsive (or, more correctly, when such responsiveness was first observed by others), a new strategy be adopted.

A view contrary to that of Perry's—namely, that active attempts at rehabilitation are both worthwhile and indicated whilst patients remain comatose—found support, at least in some US clinics, around the same time. For instance, among the contributors to a 1983 issue of the journal *Physical Therapy*, which was entirely devoted to the subject of head injury, Danese Malkmus wrote in the following terms of strategies that physical therapists might adopt in the earliest stage of recovery:

> [T]he physical therapist is in an ideal position to address not only physical management concerns, but the individual's depressed state of responsiveness. A sensory stimulation program may be constructed and taught to nursing personnel, family members and others having patient contact during the acute phase. Stimulation that may increase intracranial pressure, however, should be avoided.[3]

A caveat was added: 'Physician consultation and approval should be obtained before implementing a program.' Danese Malkmus, the author of the article, was

---

2 Jacquelin Perry (1983) Rehabilitation of the neurologically disabled patient: principles, practice and scientific basis. *Journal of Neurosurgery, 58,* 799.
3 Danese Malkmus (1983) Integrating cognitive strategies into the physical therapy setting. *Physical Therapy, 63,* 1952.

co-director of the Head Injury Center at Hyannis, USA. Significantly, Freeman visited Hyannis in 1983 during the course of development of his approach to brain injury and was impressed by the centre.

The Glasgow Coma Scale

In any study of coma, it is necessary to agree on some scale of measurement of its depth if comparisons with the observations reported by others are to become possible. Similar considerations apply to the individual patient when the attending medical personnel wish to compare examinations undertaken at different times and so formulate estimates of progress in recovery.

The Glasgow Coma Scale (GCS) was devised by two leading neurosurgeons in the United Kingdom, Professor Graham Teasdale and Professor Bryan Jennett.[4] A measurement of the depth of coma provides a baseline with which subsequent examinations could be compared. The GCS is set out in Table 4.1.

Table 4.1 The Glasgow Coma Scale

Eyes			
Open	Spontaneously	4
	To verbal command	3
	To pain	2
No response		1
Best verbal response			
	Orientated and converses	5
	Disorientated and converses	4
	Inappropriate words	3
	Incomprehensible sounds	2
	No response	1
Best motor response			
To verbal command	Obeys	6
To painful stimulus	Localises pain	5
	Flexion-withdrawal	4
	Flexion-abnormal (decorticate rigidity)	3
	Extension (decerebrate rigidity)	2
	No response	1
Total		3–15

Source: Bryan Jennett & Graham Teasdale (1974) Assessment of coma and impaired consciousness. *The Lancet*, *ii*, 81.

---

4   Bryan Jennett & Graham Teasdale (1974) Assessment of coma and impaired consciousness. *The Lancet*, *ii*, 81.

The GCS is used throughout the world as a simple assessment measurement and the result of examining a patient can vary from 3 to 15. The factors measured in the scale are

1.   the extent of eye opening

2.   the making of sounds or words

3.   movement in response to touch or pain or voice.

The lowest score (3) indicates that no response has been detected to any stimulus. It may be recalled that the young patient Ian, whose case notes were included in Chapter 2, was scored at three. Patients who are assessed at 8 or below are regarded as being in coma and those at 9 or above are considered to have come out of coma. This does not imply that they are fully recovered—often far from it.

To be aware or not to be?

Freeman's case notes and the family stories presented above describe many occasions on which patients were referred to as being 'vegetative' and predicted to remain in this category.

The defined characteristics of the vegetative state and the persistent vegetative state (PVS) are similar. The only distinction is the duration of the state. The US Multi-Society Task Force on PVS summed it up: 'By definition, patients in PVS are unaware of themselves or their environment.'[5] An interesting example of the flexibility accorded by an adaptable acronym has been the later substitution of 'permanent' for 'persistent' in PVS with consequent implications for management. Recent initiatives to adopt a new terminology, based on observations of cerebral activity in affected patients, will be referred to below.

Notwithstanding the precise definitions attached to the vegetative state by authoritative bodies, it is very likely that the term 'vegetative' had frequently been incorrectly applied in the case of people discussed in the earlier chapters. Whether expressed as prolonged unconsciousness, coma or vegetative state, these diagnoses were frequently inaccurate in patients whom Freeman encountered, as also were the predicted outcomes.

The decision by a clinician that some level of awareness is present requires the qualification that this interpretation essentially represents the *ascertainment*, *recognition* or *detection by that clinician* of the presence of some awareness. In essence, the attachment of the diagnosis to any patient reflects not only the

---

5   Multi-Society Task Force on PVS (1994) Medical aspects of the persistent vegetative state. Part 1. *New England Journal of Medicine, 330*, 1499.

actual condition of that patient but also the capacity of the clinical observer to recognise this. Awareness is required on the part of both patient and clinician if it is to be diagnosed. Awareness on the part of the patient is not necessarily accompanied by comparable ability on his or her part to indicate its presence to another individual.

The neural apparatus necessary for awareness and that required for a patient to be able to demonstrate awareness to others are discrete. The former may remain intact whilst the latter is disabled. This occurs typically in individuals who are diagnosed as 'locked in'. Signs that an aware but immobile person can give may be detectable only by some observers and be manifest only inconsistently. It would hardly be surprising if a locked-in person became extremely frustrated by his or her predicament, a response likely to be manifest in aggressive behaviour.

In the same way that awareness and the capacity to demonstrate its existence to others are not necessarily coexistent, nor are the ability to experience something and the ability to remember it. The discrete nature of experience and memory in individuals who appear to be unconscious has been known for half a century, following the first report by Bernard Levinson of retained awareness by patients under general anaesthesia.[6] A large volume of research subsequently on the subject of awareness under general anaesthesia (aided and abetted by legal proceedings instituted by aggrieved patients) has validated its occurrence.

In the circumstances of anaesthetic practice, amnesia was a consequence of ancillary medication. There is, however, nothing to exclude the likelihood that traumatic brain damage in some people may compromise memory to a greater extent than occurs with awareness. Meeting an individual who has regained consciousness and is able to provide an account of events that occurred in the vicinity while in coma provides impressive testimony to awareness retained whilst comatose. That another person, after regaining consciousness, is unable to match this performance does not exclude the possibility that she or he may have had similar experience, albeit not remembered.

Freeman's experience that the diagnosis of 'vegetative' was often not accurate at the time when he met a patient was entirely consistent with conclusions that were increasingly being reported throughout the 1970s and 1980s by clinicians outside Australia.

Whilst the vegetative state was believed to be an entity that could be diagnosed with great certainty, this was becoming increasingly acknowledged not to be so in the early 1990s by some clinicians. A misdiagnosis rate of 37 per cent was reported by Nancy Childs and colleagues among patients referred to a

---

6   Bernard Levinson (1965) States of awareness under general anaesthesia. *British Journal of Anaesthesia,* *37,* 544.

hospital in Texas.[7] The American Congress of Rehabilitation Medicine released a statement in 1995 to the effect that knowledge of misdiagnosis of the condition was longstanding, and added, ominously, that the situation was not improving.[8] Probably the most influential statement of the situation in the 1990s, reflecting its publication in a widely read journal, was that of Keith Andrews and colleagues. They reported that 17 of 40 patients referred by specialists to the Royal Hospital for Neurodisability with a diagnosis of PVS were not vegetative.[9] While it might be contended that these patients had regained consciousness after the original diagnosis was made, the history of 'prolonged coma' in all cases renders this an unlikely explanation.

Among the people whom he met who were definitely not vegetative, Freeman considered some to be 'locked in'. The locked-in syndrome was originally described as an entity with well-defined neuropathological features, and clinical signs corresponding to these, by Fred Plum and Jerome Posner in 1966.[10] That original pathological categorisation of affected individuals held that the cerebral cortex remained intact (permitting awareness) but that neural pathways had been interrupted by damage to the brain stem. Subsequently, it was discovered that the pathological features of locked-in patients could be quite diverse and that there was not necessarily a close correspondence between pathological anatomy and clinical features.[11]

Underlying the diagnostic approach to an apparently comatose person that Freeman developed in the course of practice has been a longstanding concern that the patient may actually be aware although unable to communicate with the examining practitioner—that is, in a locked-in condition as noted above. A quite compelling concern about this was well expressed in a 1980 paper from an Italian neurosurgical clinic:

> There always remains some lingering doubt that the patient may have some mental activity which we have simply failed to detect. This doubt is often kindled by claims from those caring for the vegetative wreck on a full time basis that the patient actually makes himself understood in some uncommon or even eerie way.[12]

7   Nancy L. Childs, Walt N. Mercer & Helen W. Childs (1993) Accuracy of diagnosis of persistent vegetative state. *Neurology, 43*, 1465.

8   American Congress of Rehabilitation Medicine (1995) Recommendations for use of uniform nomenclature pertinent to patients with severe alterations in consciousness. *Archives of Physical Medicine and Rehabilitation, 76*, 205.

9   Keith Andrews, Lesley Murphy, Ros Munday & Clare Littlewood (1996) Misdiagnosis of the vegetative state: retrospective study in a rehabilitation unit. *British Medical Journal, 1313*, 13.

10   Fred Plum & Jerome Posner (1966) *The Diagnosis of Stupor and Coma*. F. A. Davis, Philadelphia.

11   Joseph S. Karp & Howard I. Hurtig (1974) 'Locked-in' state with bilateral mid brain infarcts. *Archives of Neurology, 30*, 176; James R. Patterson & Martin Grabois (1986) Locked-in syndrome: a review of 139 cases. *Stroke, 17*, 758.

12   Albino Bricolo, Sergio Trazzi & Giannantonio Feriotti (1980) Prolonged post-traumatic unconsciousness. Therapeutic assets and liabilities. *Journal of Neurosurgery, 52*, 625.

Freeman's success in often detecting indications of awareness when others had been unable to do so may be attributed to at least two factors. First, his manner of approaching the patient and his patience in undertaking a slow and sometimes unorthodox clinical examination seem to be central. Second, his preparedness to accord value to the observations of laypersons who had spent prolonged periods with the patient, usually his or her family. This practice of involving the family extended, whenever possible, to his examination of the patient and could lead to detection of signs of awareness not conceivably detectable in a conventional clinical examination. Roger's story of response to a cartridge in Chapter 2 exemplifies this well.

A 2009 report from Joseph Giacino and colleagues, based on comparison of observations from rehabilitation clinics and the Cyclotron Research Centre at the University of Liege, drew attention to the disparity between the results of neuro-imaging of unconscious patients and conclusions based on their conventional clinical examination. Having made the point that clinical diagnosis of coma depends upon observation of the patient's behaviour, the authors emphasised the potential, frequently realised, for misdiagnosis to occur. The factors underlying diagnostic variance between clinical assessment and the results of neuro-imaging (invariably entailing the detection of cerebral activity by imaging when clinical examination failed to do so) were classified by the authors into three categories relating to the examiner, the patient and the environment.

The examining clinician may sample too narrow a range of behaviour, or examine too infrequently and use poorly defined criteria for judging purposeful responsiveness. The patient may have a fluctuating level of arousal, be fatigued and have motor impairment that curtails attempts to respond. Environmental obstacles could include sedation, poor positioning and restraint restricting the patient's range of movement.[13]

The frequent disparity observed between clinical and imaging examination of patients led, in a 2010 article from Liege, to a proposal for a change in nomenclature to describe patients in prolonged coma. Having commented on the pejorative connotations implicit in the application of a description as 'vegetative', Steven Laureys and his colleagues continued:

> [M]oreover, since its first description over 35 years ago, an increasing number of functional neuroimaging and cognitive evoked potential studies have shown that physicians should be cautious to make strong claims about awareness in some patients without behavioural responses to command.

---

13   Joseph T. Giacino, Caroline Schnakers, Diana Rodriquez-Moreno, Kathy Kalmar, Nicholas Schiff & Joy Hirsch (2009) Behavioural assessment in patients with disorders of consciousness: gold standard or fool's gold? *Progress in Brain Research, 177,* 177.

The authors suggested that the expression 'vegetative state' could advantageously be replaced with another: 'unresponsive wakefulness syndrome.'[14]

Another article from Liege, published in the following year, expanded on the revised nomenclature and the reasons for it:

> Some severely brain damaged patients may show residual cortical processing in the absence of behavioural signs of consciousness. Given these new findings, the diagnostic errors and their potential effects on treatment as well as concerns regarding the negative associations intrinsic to the term vegetative state, the European Task Force on Disorders of Consciousness has recently proposed the more neutral and descriptive term unresponsive wakefulness syndrome. When vegetative/unresponsive patients show minimal signs of consciousness but are unable to communicate reliably the term minimally responsive or minimally conscious state (MCS) is used.[15]

Freeman's concept, to be discussed below, of a 'fragile period' during which (soft) signs of awareness may be inconsistently detectable led to difficulties, and criticism, when attempts were made to conduct a clinical trial of his procedures. This trial will be discussed below. Nevertheless, as with many of the practices for which he attracted criticism in Australia, his thinking was close to that of respected overseas practitioners. For instance, the statement that '[f]amily members and others with whom the patient has a close relationship may be able to obtain a response when others have failed' could have been written by him but was actually suggested by two rehabilitation specialists at the Greenery Rehabilitation and Skilled Nursing Center in Boston.[16]

Freeman's account of his life in Chapter 1 recalls the sequence of events that inexorably led to his career commitment of trying to assist people most of whom had been classified ominously as 'not suitable for rehabilitation' following brain injury. One of these events, which appears to have been very influential in his later work, was his observation of the extreme care and consideration shown by some experienced and humane US practitioners towards children with severe neurological and mental disabilities. This contrasted with his dismay when he was personally confronted with the 'mass production warehousing' of many other children in this category at Peat Island. This consisted, as he has described

---

14   Steven Laureys, Gastone G. Celesia, Jan Lavrijsen, Jose Leon-Carrion, Walter G. Sannita, Leon Sazbon, Erich Schumutzhard, Klaus R. van Wild, Adam Zeman & Guiliano Dolce (2010) Unresponsive wakefulness syndrome: a new name for the vegetative state or apallic syndrome. *BMC Medicine, 1*, 68.

15   Marie-Aurelie Bruno, Audrey Vanhaudenhuyse, Aurore Thibaut, Gustave Moonen & Steven Laureys (2011) From unresponsive wakefulness to minimally conscious PLUS and functional locked-in syndromes: recent advances in our understanding of disorders of consciousness. *Journal of Neurology, 258*, 1373.

16   John Whyte & Mel B. Glenn (1986) The care and rehabilitation of the patient in a persistent vegetative state. *Journal of Head Trauma Rehabilitation, 1*, 1.

earlier, of little more than feeding and cleaning of a patient with minimal other human contact and scant regard for privacy, accompanied by environmental deprivation.

An episode that seems to have especially impressed him was the occasion when he observed an American physician, Edward Le Winn, who had practised at the Albert Einstein Medical Center in Philadelphia. Freeman has described this experience:

> *Dr Le Winn examined children with severe brain injury. He took his time when speaking to the patient and the parents, and he carried out the clinical examination and assessment with great sensitivity and gentleness. Whether Le Winn was correct or not in his method of assessment I couldn't say, but at least he had an approach. This seemed better than the traditional attitude of doing nothing for these children except admitting them to institutions. During lunch I spoke with the parents and their children. The parents appeared to be normal and realistic people, but there was certainly evidence of hope that something could be achieved for their children.*

The family role

The crucial role that families played, under Freeman's direction, in recovery from severe brain injuries will have been evident already in the preceding chapters. This family role commenced from the time of injury and took the form of ongoing advocacy accompanying continuing attendance at the patient's bedside. During the period of unconsciousness, Freeman noted:

> *The families seemed to have a common story. They had the greatest admiration for the way the intensive care staff had treated their patient and the care given by the neurosurgeons, but they told me the moment the patient was transferred from the intensive care unit to the high-dependency ward, they noticed an enormous drop in the amount of attention being given. They said that in their opinion it appeared that the patient was being 'parked', as if waiting for him or her to wake up.*

The presence of family members at the bedside of an unresponsive patient with a brain injury is likely to provide an environment that is beneficial. The clinical exploitation of the power of environmental stimuli with particular relevance for the rehabilitation of unconscious children was advocated in a 2009 report on the basis of observations from experiments with animals.[17] Having drawn attention to the efficacy of environmental enrichment in promoting neural plasticity and positive functional outcomes when tested in animal models, Paul Penn and colleagues advocated their application to rehabilitation of children with brain injuries.

An indication, based on electrical responses recorded from the patient's brain, provides objective support for the importance of stimuli with specific relevance to the patient. A 2008 report from a Lyon hospital described the electrical responses in the brain to speaking the specific patient's name. The patients under examination had remained unconscious for an average period of 20 days following brain injury. In a number of these patients, a unique response was observed to their name.[18] All but one of these patients had awakened when assessed three months after brain injury.

It was inferred that exposure to an individual's name could activate higher-level cognitive functions in some apparently unconscious patients. The authors concluded that, in these individuals, 'unconsciously perceived stimuli are processed and activate brain areas similarly to consciously perceived' stimuli. Furthermore, observation of response to the patient's own name could increase the prognostic value, for awakening, of electrical studies undertaken in the absence of this stimulus.

Any possibility that a family might have gained information that remained inaccessible to medical personnel, presaging a lessening of coma, would often have been discounted in medical assessment. In some instances, information from this source would be disparaged as coming from untrained observers whose interpretation had been coloured by unrealistic hopes of recovery. Disparagement sometimes extended from the families to Freeman's ideas and ultimately to him as a person. The essential role for patients' families envisaged by Freeman in a proposed clinical trial became a source of dispute with hospital personnel. It was asserted that the study could be better controlled and its results interpreted if the family role was undertaken by healthcare workers who would employ a uniform stimulation protocol.

The 'traditional' medical approach to the person who failed to wake up within a few weeks after brain injury as summarised by Freeman, and his attitude towards this, was as follows:

17 Paul Penn, David Rose & David Johnson (2009) Virtual enriched environments in paediatric neuropsychological rehabilitation following traumatic brain injury. *Developmental Rehabilitation, 12,* 32.
18 Catherine Fischer, Frederic Daillier & Dominique Morlet (2008) Novelty P3 elicited by the subject's own name in comatose patients. *Clinical Neurophysiology, 119,* 224.

> *The traditional medical approach has been to say that the coma has ended when the patient is able to obey a command.[19] But many doctors only consider the patient to be out of coma when he or she can consistently obey a command. I regard this requirement as a 'hard' sign and I question whether this is an accurate method of assessment. This need for a 'hard' sign often causes conflict between the families and the medical profession. The families and friends often observe 'soft' signs, which may be a head movement or a movement of an arm or finger or leg or a vocal sound or eye contact or a facial expression. These signs may be inconsistently present. Sometimes the doctors discount these 'soft' signs, but nevertheless they are very real to the families.*

Freeman's conclusion that signs of returning consciousness may only be inconsistently observed during the early stages of emergence (characterised by him as 'soft signs') did not sit comfortably with the generally accepted idea that only clear-cut signs that could be reproducibly identified at any time by different observers were acceptable as evidence. The concept of 'soft signs' could not readily be accommodated within a formal study of emergence—one of a number of obstacles to a trial of coma arousal. As has happened with a number of his conclusions, drawn from empirical observations, his description of 'soft signs' during emergence has recently been underpinned by a study from a Mississippi rehabilitation centre.

When introducing the report of this study, the authors note: 'Published guidelines for defining the 'minimally conscious state' (MCS) included behaviours that characterise emergence, specifically 'reliable and consistent' functional interactive communication (accurate yes/no responding) and functional use of objects.'[20]

They note that guidelines had been derived by consensus rather than on the basis of extensive data collection. In their study, some 300 patients were submitted to weekly examinations, repeated on four occasions. Consistent responses were not obtained from many patients in the early stages of emergence. In the light of this it was concluded that '[c]onsistent yes/no accuracy is uncommon among responsive patients in early recovery from TBI (traumatic brain injury). These results suggest that the operational threshold for yes/no response accuracy as a diagnostic criterion for emergence should be revisited.'

Freeman has given an account of the conventional examination of a comatose patient:

---

19   Editorial (1981) Outcome of traumatic coma. *The Lancet, ii*, 507.
20   Risa Nakase-Richardson, Stuart Yablon, Mark Sherer, Clea C. Evans & Todd G. Nick (2008) Serial yes/no reliability after traumatic brain injury: implications regarding the operational criteria for emergence from the minimally conscious state. *Journal of Neurology, Neurosurgery and Psychiatry, 79*, 216.

Often the medical assessment of a patient is like this. Accompanied by the nurse and other staff members, the clinician enters the patient's room. The clinician questions the nurse as to any changes in the condition of the patient, then checks the patient's chin, arm and leg reflexes with a small hammer. He then scratches the sole of the patient's foot to see if the big toe moves up or down. It usually moves up with severe brain injury. He squeezes the patient's calf muscles, exerting enough pressure to cause some pain, and the patient's whole body moves. The clinician is then likely to comment, 'Still showing signs of severe brain injury!' He feels the arm and leg muscles to check if their tone (tightness) is increased or diminished by grasping the limb and moving it through its range of movement.

The patient may be 'locked in' and unable to communicate during any of this time. Other tests may be performed, but the fact that the patient is present as a person may never be acknowledged. The clinician may ask the patient to obey a command such as 'look at me' or 'move your right arm'. When the patient does not respond to this command immediately, the clinician often walks away from the bed, without realising that there is a 'lag time' in the patient with a brain injury. This lag time means that even if the patient can understand the request, he is unable to marshal the thought processes necessary to undertake the request quickly. Consequently, the clinician may have already left the room by the time the action takes place and the clinical record is noted 'no change'.

It is probable that the patients discussed in the two preceding chapters had been formally assessed in a manner similar to Freeman's description above. It would conform with attitudes to brain injury prevalent in the 1980s. Whereas this strategy more or less placed the burden of proof of any retained or regained awareness on the patient, Freeman's approach was to transfer this burden onto the examining practitioner, assisted by family members. This obliged the observer to seek evidence of awareness, perhaps 'soft signs' that could not be consistently demonstrated, and to give credence to family-sourced descriptions of these, which were to be followed up. In the case of patients for whom no family members were accessible, Freeman's strategy was severely restricted.

Accompanying the 'conventional' medical position that a regular neurological examination would suffice to exclude the possibility of retained or regained awareness was the belief that all participants, other than the patient, were spectators of any recovery process. It followed that any attempts to assist or to expedite the return of awareness were, by definition, pointless.

Freeman's observations on what *was* done with patients who remained comatose after brain injury and his thoughts on what *could* be done led him to develop an examination protocol. His description of this follows:

When assessing a patient in coma I took a totally different approach to the clinical method described above. I took the view that the family was my most priceless resource for they provided the loving bridge that enabled me to gain information about the patient and I found them to be extremely reliable. This approach is not new. I was taught this in medical school. Sir Lorimer Dodds, a superb clinician and the Senior Physician at the Royal Alexandra Hospital for Children in Sydney, taught us to observe these maxims when assessing a child who cannot speak for himself—'Always listen to the mother … It is a foolish doctor who does not take notice of what the mother says … More things in medicine are missed by not looking rather than not knowing.'

Three important aspects that he regarded as critical in the way in which he approached the examination of any patient were characterised as the 'fragile period', the 'approach distance' and the 'mantle of safety'. Freeman has described the origins of his concept of the 'fragile period':

After studying the Glasgow Coma Scale, like many others, I soon realised that the measuring components of eye opening and the making of sounds had problems. Often, to measure eye opening was invalid because the patient had injuries to the eyes or to the nerves of the eye, and the making of sounds was often impossible as a tube had been inserted through the vocal cords into the trachea.

I consider the most important steps in the assessment of returning awareness is first measured by the reaction of the patient to touch and pain, two of the most fundamental sensations. This regaining of awareness can be charted using the following method:

1. No response to pain places the patient at the lower end of the scale.

2. A reflex response whether of extension (straightening) or flexion (bending) of an arm or leg in response to a painful stimulus being applied is the next step up.

3. The reaction of withdrawal of the limb or body from pain stimulus.

4. Localising to a painful or touch stimulus places the person at a higher level of response again. (Localising means that when a stimulus is applied to a part of the body, the eyes and/or head will turn to that stimulus or the hand will move towards it.)

5. Discrimination—at the highest level, occurs when the brain picks up the stimulus and begins to recognise it.

I have called the period B-C, between initial awareness and 'normal' awareness, the 'fragile period'.

Figure 4.1 The 'Fragile Period'

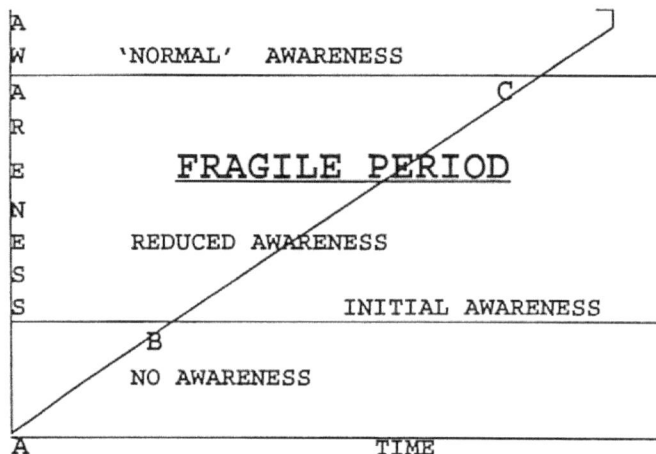

The period A-B theoretically and for practical purposes indicates the vegetative state or an absolute and total 'locked-in state'. During this time there is no evidence of any reaction to a stimulus. Obviously, many patients pass through this stage before they reach a point of initial awareness or move out of the 'locked-in state'.

C indicates the obeying of a command. This passage from B to C through the fragile period must be like a person looking up from the bottom of a swimming pool. At the bottom, all is blurred and familiar objects such as the pool steps are difficult to recognise. As the swimmer moves closer to the surface, objects become more distinct and recognisable. It is similar with the person arousing from coma. The patient may have some awareness but in the early stages it is vague and unclear. This fragile period also means that because the person has some awareness he can be emotionally hurt by insensitive comments at the bedside and by painful treatments. The person may also be aware that his personal space has been violated by nasogastric tubes and tracheostomy tubes, and it is very likely that the person is in a state of sensory deprivation.

The patient, while considered by some members of the medical profession to have no awareness, may have a significant amount of awareness. In my opinion, this passage from initial awareness to the conscious state can be clarified by close observation. The families who have spent time with the person they love and have observed the 'soft' signs are the ones who can generally indicate to the doctor when the patient has begun to travel up through these definite levels of awareness. Other specific indicators of awareness are the facial expressions of the patients, which when appropriate to the environment can demonstrate consciousness—for example, smiling when jokes are told, anxiety at unpleasant experiences, sadness when families indicate they are leaving. These may constitute a 'cluster of soft signs'.

I am extremely conscious of the need to safeguard a person's 'approach distance', especially when that person is totally incapable of defending him/herself and will rapidly go into a stress reaction with its 'fight, freeze or flight' pattern. I am aware that the totally dependent person who can neither fight nor take flight will freeze and give the observer a mistaken impression that they are not aware when they may be fully conscious and locked in. This is especially so if the person has had gross violation of their intimate space by catheters, a tracheostomy tube, and abdominal or chest drains.

I always provided 'a mantle of safety' for the patient. This term was used by the Reverend John Flynn, founder of the Australian Inland Mission and the Royal Flying Doctor Service, when referring to the isolation and lack of support for people living in the Australian outback.

Freeman's account of the examination process was as follows:

To start an assessment, I always met with the family in a room away from the patient and sat down with them to explore what they had observed in the patient. I explained that they were not in a court of law and did not all have to agree on what they had seen or felt. I pointed out that if the patient was truly vegetative none of them would have seen any normal reactions. I also pointed out that if the patient was aware then he would react more to them than to any other person since he would know that they were his loved ones, and they as family would be infinitely more aware of the patient's reactions than any doctor or nurse, since they were the ones who knew him best and were spending far more time with him than any professional could.

A very structured set of questions was developed by Freeman to present to family members:

1. Vigilance: Why do you believe the patient is awake? Does he know you are present? Why do you think that? Does he react to different people in the family? Does he react to one nurse more than the others? Does he react when his environment is changed?

2. Emotion: Does he show facial expressions indicating anxiety, fear, anger, pleasure, disgust, and so on? Is this appropriate? For example, does he show sadness and have tears in his eyes as you say you are about to leave? Does he show fear when the suction apparatus is switched on? (The suction in these patients is often carried out by a long plastic tube introduced into the endotracheal tube, which has been placed in the trachea. The tip of the sucker often hits the tracheal wall and causes a great deal of coughing and distress to the patient. If the patient shows fear when it is turned on it also indicates he has memory and anticipation. Both are higher cortical functions of the brain. Sometimes other apparatus such as the floor polisher can cause a similar sound to the suction tube and the patient may react in a similar way, showing fear.)

3. Drive: Can you get any actions from the patient by asking him? No matter how slight the actions, can they be repeated?

I then ask about the senses of vision, hearing, touch, taste and smell before moving on to asking what the patient can do with movement of the head, body, arms, hands and legs, and so on. I always allowed enough time for all the family members to put forward their personal views.

Some of my colleagues viewed everything the families said and all their positive offerings as 'wishful thinking' or 'unreal hope', but I found most families to be enormously truthful, honest and realistic. Their observations, made over many hours of sitting with the patient, provided me with valuable information, which then gave me an excellent idea of whether the patient was showing signs of awareness or not, and what the patient could and could not do. In my experience, rarely did a family member report observations that were obviously exaggerated or impossible.

In an inquiring and prolonged manner, I gathered the details needed for my assessment protocol. When it was time for me to examine the patient I always asked the two closest members of the family to go into the patient and state the following: 'Doctor Freeman is coming in to see you. We will be with you for all the time he is here. He will not hurt you. He will tell you beforehand if he is going to touch you.' By this method, I surrounded the patient with people who loved him and would ensure that nothing would be done to hurt him. This took away the 'inward flight' and allowed the patient to open like a flower.

Upon entering the room, I introduced myself to the patient: 'My name is Ted Freeman. I will tell you if I am going to touch you. I will not hurt you.' Often I would ask the patient, 'Would you like to shake hands?' I would stretch out my own hand. It was amazing how frequently the so-called vegetative patient would attempt to reach out for my hand. I would never do anything to the patient until I had first asked a member of the family to carry out a series of tests. I would tell them what to do and I observed the reactions of the patient.

Fortuitously, Freeman's regular practice of using a family member as a 'proxy', if at all practicable, when physical contact with a patient was to occur, enabled him to undertake a worthwhile examination on those occasions when he had only been permitted to visit by the medical 'custodians' on condition that he was not to touch the patient. In more extreme examples of custody, Freeman was precluded from visiting the patient. His account continued:

Almost invariably at the end of my time with the patient, often in excess of three hours, the family would say in surprise: 'No doctor has ever sat with us before and asked us those questions or sought our opinion like you have.' Or: 'You are the only doctor we have met who seemed to know what to do.' It was by using the families as the bridge to the patient, by learning of their knowledge and by using an extended assessment time that the true state of the patient could be properly gauged. After nearly 20 years of involvement with patients diagnosed as PVS, my estimate is that approximately 90 per cent of those patients showed evidence of awareness and were not vegetative.

In each stage we found that the families were more skilled at identifying responses to a stimulus because of the bond of trust and love that existed between themselves and the patient.

We also found that other factors could have an important bearing on the patient's response to a stimulus, such as the time of the day: generally patients responded better in the morning than the evening. Constipation and also the febrile state could cause the patient to feel listless, causing the responses to vary, as could the failure of a good rapport between the assessor and the patient. But these factors tended to be difficult to quantify and qualify.

The Coma Exit Chart

Whilst the GCS is a valuable way of assessing the depth of any patient's coma, Freeman believed that it lacked the sensitivity necessary to detect very early indications of awareness. This may not have been a concern if the treating practitioner adhered to the belief that everyone caring for the patient was a spectator witnessing an event the progression of which they had no ability to influence. On the other hand, if one believed that the possibility existed of favourably influencing the rate and ultimate extent of that progression then the availability of some method to monitor it would be a powerful ancillary tool in assisting both. On any assessment, Freeman deserves credit for initiating the development of a strategy to monitor emergence, especially when this was slow and irregular. He developed the Coma Exit Chart, described as follows:

> With an input from the observations of families of patients, together with my own observations, I formulated the 'Coma Exit Chart'. This chart has been modified in the United Kingdom to form the Sensory Modality Assessment Rehabilitation and Treatment (SMART) tool.[21]

Commenting on the value of the chart and the study preceding it, Dr Sarah Wilson, Senior Lecturer in the Department of Psychological Medicine of the University of Glasgow, wrote:

> As a psychologist with over twenty years' experience of working with individuals who have suffered very severe brain injury including those with a diagnosis of vegetative state, I have found Dr Freeman's work to be an invaluable contribution to helping both patients and their families.

> I have recommended both his books *The Catastrophe of Coma: A Way Back* and *Brain Injury & Stroke: A Handbook to Recovery* to colleagues and patients' relatives. I routinely incorporate Dr Freeman's Coma Exit Chart in my assessment of patients diagnosed as being in a vegetative state (including use within a medico-legal context) and I regularly recommend its use to colleagues. Dr Freeman is recognised internationally for his expertise. His work has generated further research and is undoubtedly of benefit to patients with severe brain injury.[22]

The Coma Exit Chart has exerted a significant influence on the development of a tool for assessment of comatose patients in many overseas clinics. Thus, Dr Keith Andrews, Director of Medical and Research Services, Royal Hospital for Neurodisability, London, has written:

> Dr Freeman has made a considerable contribution to the understanding of, and attitude to, people with profound brain damage, especially those in the vegetative state. His book *The Catastrophe of Coma* has been recommended by us to numerous relatives of patients in the vegetative state and they have found it illuminating, practical and supportive. Dr Freeman's work was the stimulation and basis of our research into

---

21 Edward Freeman (1993) The clinical assessment of coma. *Neuropsychological Rehabilitation, 3*, 139; Edward Freeman (1996) New methodology. The coma exit chart: assessing the patient in prolonged coma and the vegetative state. *Brain Injury, 10*, 615.
22 Sarah Wilson, Letter to Freeman, April 2002.

the vegetative state and the development of the Sensory Modality Assessment Rehabilitation and Treatment tool (SMART) which is now the standard for assessment in brain damage in the UK.[23]

Other modifications and refinements have followed—for example, an Italian version has been developed, written by the lead author of the Cochrane Review of coma arousal reports, which will be considered later when discussing a clinical trial of Freeman's procedures.[24]

To conclude this account of Freeman's approach to improving the situation of comatose patients, it is appropriate to quote from an article in which he listed six major changes that he advocated. These concerned both the practices of clinicians managing individual patients and the manner in which the healthcare system could improve their condition:

1. Trial of therapy

In an effort to increase the level of awareness of the patient, I would advocate a trial of therapy. Trials of therapy are common in medicine when the outcome of the disease process and the optimum type of treatment are unknown.

In this course of action the disease process is first defined and the therapy, whether drug or physical therapy, is applied for a trial of weeks or months or longer to observe whether it has changed the likely outcome. During this time the patient is closely monitored to ensure there are no disadvantageous events.

Since the patient with severe brain injury is in a state of sensory and emotional deprivation, a structured input of sensory stimuli can be devised for each person depending upon their position on the SMART test.

Emotional deprivation must be regarded as a constant state, and monitoring of the stimuli must be continuous to ensure that the maximum amount of positive stimulation is given. Negative stimuli are inherent in a hospital environment and often an essential part of the treatment. Steps should be taken to make certain that unnecessary negative stimuli are reduced to a minimum.

2. Coma Care Units

A Coma Care Unit is the optimum place in which to conduct the trial of therapy. These units should be similar to coronary care units, intensive care

23   Keith Andrews, Letter to Freeman, May 2002.
24   Francesco Lombardi, Giordano Gatta, Simona Sacco, Anna Muratori & Antonia Carolei (2007) The Italian version of the coma recovery scale revised. *Functional Neurology, 22,* 47.

units, burns units, spinal units etc. This would allow intensive research into the process of the arousal from coma and the problems of treatment, with protocols automatically undergoing change and improvement as the knowledge of brain injury increases.

Since the long term costs of severe brain injury are high, the gains made with the increasing knowledge about patient response and outcomes would offset these costs.

3. Coma Register

The patients and the medical profession would benefit from a Coma Register. Since no one knows how many patients survive severe brain injury or remain in coma two weeks post trauma, it is essential to know the size of the problem. (Two weeks in coma is a marker time of great importance since it was (is) considered that the outcome of the injury is likely to be poor).

4. Coma Care Review Committee

At the time of notification to the register, a special committee called the Coma Care Review Committee consisting of both professionals and relatives (if available) would assess the patient and then monitor the treatment and progress of the patient. The flow of patients from the Coma Care Unit would be to home for domiciliary rehabilitation if possible, otherwise to a Special Facility. The decision making process at this point would be the responsibility of the Coma Care Review Committee in conjunction with family members.

5. Special Facility for Patients Diagnosed as 'Locked In' or Vegetative

There will always be patients who demonstrate awareness but fail to progress or do so very slowly and are classified as in the 'locked in' state. It is important to have a suitable facility for provision of their needs. Every effort must be made to initiate muscle function and improve communication so they can gain a level of independence and make known their needs and wants. A constant process of monitoring to change programs will be required.

6. Long Term Review Committee

It is essential that a Long Term Review Committee be established so that the people in the Special Facility are not cut adrift from the medical and educational systems. They should be assessed by knowledgeable people at set intervals or on request. If there are signs of improvement a new program should be structured to suit their particular needs.[25]

Conclusion

Ted Freeman has made a significant contribution to understanding the process of regaining consciousness following brain injury and to the clinical recognition of that process. This contribution was largely based on two practices—namely, paying attention to the observations reported by patients' families, and developing a strategy for patient examination that provided the best environment for detecting early signs of awakening.

In order to afford the best chance of gleaning information about a patient's current status, Freeman used an exhaustive protocol for questioning family members. This drew his attention to manifestations of awakening that were observed only inconsistently, which he described as 'soft signs'. Recognition and acceptance of the importance of these soft signs stimulated the development of his Coma Exit Chart, which facilitated documentation of awakening from coma and so complemented what the Glasgow Coma Scale had done for assessing the depth of coma.

Freeman's insights into unconsciousness occurred at a time when there was increasing recognition internationally that misdiagnosis of the vegetative state—attributable to failure to detect subtle signs of consciousness—was common. Because he paid considerable attention to the reported observations of 'untrained observers'—namely, patients' family members—and because he spent prolonged periods examining patients, with assistance from family members, many of his colleagues rejected his conclusions. Recently, objective evidence supporting many of his conclusions has become available as a result of refinements in scanning of brain activity. These include recognition of brain activity in patients diagnosed as unconscious and the salience of environmental cues with personal significance in eliciting brain activity. An approach to assessing Freeman's impact on clinical practice is described in Chapter 8.

---

25   Edward Freeman (1992) The persistent vegetative state—the fate worse than death. *Clinical Rehabilitation*, 6,159.

5. What future after emergence?

This chapter's primary aim is to describe the development and implementation of Freeman's ideas for assisting patients and their families through the period after discharge from an acute-care hospital. What it was possible to achieve in practice evolved through several stages, largely as a result of the changing circumstances within which he practised. The intersection between Freeman's life and his fight on behalf of his patients, referred to above, is most evident in this chapter.

Freeman's absolute horror at the plight of those who had been effectively abandoned within the healthcare system, with no possibility of ongoing rehabilitation, was clearly a strong motivating influence for him. He has provided an account of a visit to Weemala, an institution which held a significant number of younger people with long-term severe brain injuries. This visit occurred in 1989, a decade after his initial commitment to the research, but it is likely to represent an accurate summary of his impressions following earlier visits to similar institutions. It is, incidentally, an indication that not much had changed by this later date.

The visit in question was undertaken to assess a young man with a severe brain injury, at the request of his parents. Freeman found that one in eight of the residents was there on account of brain injury. Perhaps these were part of the group who had no family support. Perhaps they included people like Cecil, in Chapter 2, whose family had acted on the advice to 'walk away and forget'. There are also likely to have been patients without families and others whose families lacked the resources, including financial capacity, required to care for them at home. He reports that:

> Weemala smelt of despair and when I visited there I felt that I was back in Ward Four at Peat Island. There was a scarcity of staff and few visitors. There was no noise except for the heart-wrenching cries of the inmates tied in their beds or chairs. The place was filled with bad odours, which could be detected the moment you entered the building. Weemala had been built in 1906 for Sir Henry Moses and had been bequeathed by him as a Home for Incurables. In 1989 it had 176 patients. Twenty of these were admitted with severe brain injury. There were patients with stroke, multiple sclerosis, cerebral palsy, cerebral tumours, mental retardation and rheumatoid arthritis. The wards varied from two to seven beds. There was limited privacy, provided by yellow curtains hanging from rails around each bed. There was no area for the patients' special belongings, and in the

hospital brochure it states, 'Valuable items and large sums of money are best left at home or in a bank safe deposit, no responsibility can be accepted for lost or stolen goods.'

I found Weemala repulsive, and mentally cleansed myself when I had finished my inspection, appalled by what I had witnessed and outraged that any person should be subjected to such suffering, and certainly not those whom the minister responsible for Weemala called 'helpless people'. If this was protection by legislation, the legislation urgently needed to be revised.

Freeman's observations on Weemala describe a situation in which virtually all of the practical initiatives provided to patients in the course of his ideal post-emergence rehabilitation scenario were countermanded. Sensory input was denied by the system. Any 'risk' of stimulation was minimised. Inadequate staffing precluded any attempt to provide some opportunity for interaction between a resident and another person, even if this had been institutional policy, which it clearly was not.

At the same time, staff limitations would minimise chances of any manifestation of 'soft signs' being reported, let alone acted upon, again even if this had been policy. The conditions were certainly dissuasive of visitors and, even if some had ventured in, would have precluded attempts to undertake any program.

As recounted in Chapter 1, Freeman's consuming interest in the plight of people who had remained unconscious beyond the acute stage of brain injury and his resulting interaction with unorthodox therapists led to the termination of his appointment at Peat Island. An opportunity to remain committed to the management of affected people was provided, in the first instance, by the offer of financial support from World Vision and then by an undertaking on the part of the NSW Government Insurance Office (GIO) to provide support. As part of this agreement, Freeman became Medical Director of the newly formed Brain Injury Division of the Australian Brain Foundation.

Under this new arrangement, his first opportunity to apply on a larger scale the practices that he had come to recommend for individual patients came with the provision of funding to trial those practices on a group of inpatients. This trial was to occur in the Westmead Hospital. The story of the failure of the trial to proceed will be considered in the next chapter but it may be noted at this stage that a refusal by his colleagues to accept the continuity of the rehabilitation process beyond awakening and on to subsequent management was a substantial obstacle. Nevertheless, the feasibility study preparatory to the trial was completed and served a useful purpose in extending practical knowledge of both opportunities and difficulties.

With the abandonment of the 'Westmead' project, the GIO withdrew funding from the hospital. In place of it, the GIO provided funding to support the implementation of Freeman's rehabilitation strategies in a freestanding inpatient facility, the Brain Injury Therapy Centre (BITC). The period of operation of the BITC—a little more than three years—permitted the enthusiastic application of the full gamut of his ideas for ongoing rehabilitation. This period provides the source of the approaches to be described below.

The functioning of the BITC was irrevocably curtailed in 1989 as a consequence of a violent assault on the Centre and on Freeman by the NSW Minister for Health. This assault, under the protection of parliamentary privilege, represented the culmination of an ongoing attack that took a variety of forms. The nature of this attack, together with an examination of its basis, is the subject of Chapter 7.

Following the closure of the BITC, the final decade of Freeman's professional career was spent as a solo practitioner travelling to patients throughout New South Wales. Whilst this loss of resources prevented the vigorous team approach to rehabilitation that had been possible at the BITC, it inadvertently demonstrated what was achievable for patients with brain injury by means of a minimally resourced domiciliary rehabilitation program.

Any account of the development in Australia of attitudes to rehabilitation following brain injury will include much of the story of Ted Freeman's career. Accompanying the events identified in the preceding paragraphs were substantial changes in his personal circumstances. Within a short period following the parliamentary attack, he relinquished his source of income, with his professional reputation besmirched. Reference has already been made to the financial complications that commonly beset families of people with brain injury—for example, the reduction of income experienced by carers. The parliamentary attack had a similar effect on the Freemans. The manner in which Ted Freeman contrived to continue his mission of providing advice to families with a brain injured member will be recounted in the last part of this chapter.

The prognostic pessimism prevailing while patients are comatose frequently extends to the general perception of their future potential in the event of their emergence from coma. Depending on the opportunities that are available to people with a brain injury when they are no longer comatose, such pessimistic prognoses can readily become self-fulfilling. It would require overweening self-confidence in the healthcare system to postulate, as some have done, that the programs undertaken by families and volunteers had not significantly contributed to more worthwhile outcomes for many patients than those foreshadowed in their prognoses.

It will already have been clear that the patients whose stories were touched on in Chapter 3 were members of families who were committed to helping them. Surveying the many patients whose management had been influenced by Freeman's philosophy, all appear to have been members of such families. Reflecting the critical role of families in searching for some chance for their injured member, there were no instances of young patients without close next of kin coming to his attention. Most commonly, Freeman's assistance was sought directly by patients' families, with information about him having been disseminated on a 'word of mouth' basis. Yet severe head injuries are not restricted to people who are part of a strongly supportive family.

One may well ask, what about people who sustained a severe brain injury but lacked a committed family? While the numbers of patients falling into this category cannot be reliably ascertained, they have undoubtedly existed. It seems inevitable that some of the residents in the 'Home for Incurables', mentioned above, fell into this invisible cohort. It is also probable, given the stories of other patients with committed families, that some of those in this invisible cohort could have had better outcomes if they had been afforded similar opportunities.

The development of Freeman's ideas

Emergence from coma and improvement in a patient's condition thereafter represent two parts of a continuum. The separation of emergence and subsequent progress into separate chapters is intended to emphasise, as strongly as possible, patients' dependence, following awakening from coma, on the nature and level of support that are available thereafter. Far from being the end of a saga, emergence usually connotes the beginning of a much longer and more demanding period (both for patient and for family) of moving towards recovery.

The preceding point, while absolutely self-evident to families and friends, was not accepted by some of the prospective researchers in the Westmead trial. It was contended by some of those not familiar with Freeman's earlier outcomes that the participation of any patient in the trial should finish when emergence from coma was observed, or after 10 weeks, whichever came first. The reason for this limitation was that undertaking post-emergence procedures on patients in the trial was regarded as supplanting 'conventional' rehabilitation programs. This attitude failed to appreciate that the approach Freeman wished to test represented an alternative to the established approach to rehabilitation. He soon realised that straying onto another's patch can be hazardous.

This imposition of a cut-off point sought to place the attainment of a neat piece of publishable research ahead of the welfare of the patients whom the research was purported to benefit. It could be considered as a manifestation of an extreme form of 'medical compartmentalisation'. This entails a management structure in which each problem that the patient encounters is likely to be considered and dealt with in isolation, rather than the medical attendants being prepared to see the patient as a whole and regard management as an ongoing and uninterrupted program. This systemic inadequacy is not confined to patients with brain injury, nor is it a problem that has since been satisfactorily resolved, notwithstanding its widespread recognition.

Freeman has summarised what he regarded, at an early stage of his involvement, as the prevailing professional attitude towards the recovery process after brain injury:

> *I soon found that there was a considerable body of medical opinion that regarded coma as a sleep-like protective state. These people considered that nothing should be done to the person in coma, apart from general nursing care, during which time the brain would heal itself. Many orthodox doctors supported this theory and would not listen to opinions to the contrary.*

Scientific belief that 'nothing could be done' was supported by the dogmatic statement, included in every neuropathology textbook, that it was not possible to produce new neurons once an individual had grown beyond the perinatal period. That this statement is incorrect has been repeatedly demonstrated during the past decade. One unsubstantiated, and invariably unstated, assumption arising from extension of this proposition was that development of new neurons *must necessarily* be an integral component of recovery of the injured brain. *Ergo*, it was believed that 'no capacity to form new neurons' was synonymous with 'no capacity for recovery'. Contradicting this line of argument, Freeman's advocacy of the concept of 'neuroplasticity' based on observations of his patients was dismissed as scientifically untenable.

The location of post-emergence recovery will usually differ from that of the comatose stage (family home rather than acute-care hospital) and in the intensity of nursing and other care available. It has been acknowledged by medical personnel of high standing in the profession that there is an enormous difference between the care and treatment provided to patients in intensive care units and that available once they are moved to another hospital ward. For instance, Bryan Jennett, the Glasgow neurosurgeon jointly responsible for devising the Glasgow Coma Scale, commented on the situation as he saw it in 1997:

> While there are advocates for prolonged programs for active rehabilitation, the reality in most countries seems to be that many rehabilitationists are reluctant to accept these patients until they are showing some signs of recovery and are therefore expected to benefit from rehabilitation. As a result, most such patients either remain for long periods in acute care

settings or are transferred after a few weeks to nursing homes. Because of this, some believe that many vegetative patients do not reach their full potential for recovery.[1]

Jennett's insight, to which many of his colleagues would have subscribed, is notable for what it omitted. The seeming inevitability of transfer from acute care to a nursing home, or similar institution, reflected unawareness that slow-stream domiciliary rehabilitation was practicable and worthwhile for some patients. Ted Freeman's beliefs about the importance of longer-term maintenance of rehabilitation reflect his concept of the 'three accidents' that a person with a severe brain injury may experience.

> The 'first accident' is the initial trauma, an event that cannot be changed. The 'second accident' occurs when there is haemorrhage in the brain and the brain cells swell. I stressed the importance of the optimal environment to the recovering patient, after requiring intervention by the neurosurgeons and the intensivists. The 'third accident', in my opinion, occurs because often the patient is left with minimal therapy once they are out of the life-threatened state.

Arguing from the well-documented association between duration of coma and the quality of longer-term outcome, which deteriorated with prolongation of unconsciousness, Freeman suggested:

> Coma victims were placed in sensory deprivation by three factors: their injuries, the poor sensory input from their environment and the heavy use of sedative drugs.

His inference was that, if the period of impaired consciousness was shortened by measures such as less sedation and gradual introduction of opportunities for increased sensory input, subsequent outcomes might be improved. It remains impossible to determine with certainty whether the coincidence of duration of coma and extent of subsequent recovery reflects mere association or real causation. Does ultimate recovery depend only on the initial severity of the injury, or does prolonged coma aggravate the acutely inflicted injury? It seems probable that whichever interpretation is appropriate could vary from patient to patient. It might also suggest that testing the possibility of improvement in outcome as a result of shortening the period of coma is a very reasonable proposition.

As mentioned above, prognostic pessimism, when it leads, as it commonly does, to a retreat from intensive attention to the patient, often to something little

---

1 Bryan Jennett (1997) A quarter century of the vegetative state: an international perspective. *Journal of Head Trauma Rehabilitation, 12*, 1.

better than abandonment, will usually prove to be accurate. Whilst most of the patients' stories included in earlier chapters describe a family's rejection of the nursing home option in favour of caring for the patient at home, Cecil's story is a sad illustration of how the die can be cast when a gloomy forecast is acted upon.

An important factor in the inculcation of prognostic pessimism is undoubtedly the 'disconnect', referred to above by Jennett, between the medical attention available at the acute stage and in the long term. Neurosurgeons, for instance, may work unremittingly in the interests of an individual to save a life after head injury but, by the time this has been achieved, another injured individual has arrived at the hospital and is making a full-time demand on their skills.

While no numerical information is available on this point, one could wager with considerable confidence that none of Freeman's patients described in Chapters 2 or 3 had met up, several years later, with those medical professionals responsible for their acute care. With hindsight, had they done so, the pace of acceptance of Freeman's ideas may have been accelerated.

This possibility might have to be constrained by acknowledgment that awakening of a comatose patient, even when followed by a prolonged improvement to attain a life regarded as worthwhile by patient and family, is effectively a repudiation of the early prognosis. Medical professionals are certainly not unique in being uncomfortable if confronted with evidence that they got it wrong.

Another factor that has certainly been influential in prognostic pessimism, but as a 'back-up' to support the others, has been the translation into the case of the individual patient of the conventional wisdom (hardly the right noun, but the phrase can carry questioning connotations) about the pathological processes associated with brain injury that it is necessary to reverse or circumvent if any degree of recovery is to be achieved.

Finally, a factor of general applicability when individuals living with any major disability enter the healthcare system is the risk that professionals associated with their care may project their own opinions onto the patient. Thus, if *I* would not want to continue living if *I* were to be in a condition similar to that of the patient then I can 'reasonably' infer that he or she would reach a similar conclusion. To respond to this, there could be nothing more appropriate than Joe's response from Chapter 2: 'life goes on and I wouldn't be dead for quids.'

Freeman's approach to rehabilitation was essentially dependent on the families. Expressed succinctly in two of the family letters in an earlier chapter was the description of domiciliary rehabilitation as a combination of 'social contact' with 'physical activity'. The relative emphasis on these two components might vary with the age and gender of the patient. Given that many of Ted Freeman's patients were young males who had been physically active before their accidents, the strategy for older, less active persons might need to be tailored differently.

Significantly, but not unexpectedly, as already remarked, there are no histories, among Freeman's files, of patients who had a brain injury, but not a family. If one had sustained a brain injury and, in due course, had been assessed as not suitable for rehabilitation, early dispatch to a nursing home may have been inevitable. This 'invisible cohort' of patients could not be accorded input to any trial of coma arousal.

The evolution of Freeman's approach to assisting people severely disabled by brain injury appears to have taken place very much in parallel with his practical experience rather than being something that had been completely foreseen. It is likely to have been continuously amended in the light of that practical experience. As already stressed, Freeman's zeal to assist patients and their families was fuelled by his personal observation of the plight of those whom the system had sidelined. Added to this was his conviction, based on reading and supported by observations in some US clinics, that the phenomenon of brain plasticity was real. Whilst the term 'plasticity' was not in general use in relation to brain repair at the time, Freeman had been frequently making use of it in advocacy for change by 1983.

During the 1980s and 1990s the 'extraneous influences' on Freeman's practice were, I suggest, the complex financial ramifications of insurance compensation after severe brain injury, the ongoing proposition that a randomised control trial of his methods was *de rigueur* before they could be generally sanctioned and the equally ongoing opposition to the man and his methods on the part of some of his colleagues. It is not practicable at this distance in time to dissect the interplay between the last two influences, and to attempt to do so would serve little purpose now.

As a starting point for considering the strategies that evolved, one might identify Freeman's involvement with his patient Roger, described in Chapter 2. This occurred in the late 1970s when he was still employed at Peat Island. As he had no support available that could be directed to assisting patients outside that institution, the only help he could provide to patients and their families was to advise about rehabilitation measures that a family could undertake. He could also attempt to facilitate admission of the injured family member, when appropriate, to facilities that offered some chance of rehabilitation.

After leaving Peat Island, a departure largely determined by incompatibility between his views on rehabilitation after brain injury and those of his supervisors, Freeman lacked the resources to help patients until, at the beginning of 1983, the NSW GIO committed to support him. At this time, Freeman undertook a study tour of the United States, returning with increased enthusiasm for implementing programs of sensory stimulation after emergence from coma. Perhaps the observation that most impressed him about possible approaches to stimulation occurred when he visited the Greenery, a facility near Boston that specialised in rehabilitation following brain injury. He recalled:

> *The Greenery was a revelation. It had been opened 10 years previously. There was no morbid feel about the hospital. It was full of US initiative. They had active units that specifically dealt with patients in coma. Vigorous attempts at arousal of the patients took place in an effort to give them every chance to regain function. The Greenery had links with institutions that had high reputations such as Tufts New England Medical Centre and St Elisabeth's Hospital, a teaching affiliate of Tufts University.*

> *It fascinated me to see that their intense Coma Treatment Program used sensory stimulation in an effort to increase sensory awareness. They employed each of the five senses: smell, touch, taste, sight and sound. The staff/patient ratio at the Greenery was 1–1 and an average of four hours of therapy was given to each patient per day. This certainly seemed the way to go. The staff were extremely helpful and cooperative.*

Utilisation of all five senses in attempts to gain access to a patient seems quite logical if one takes account of human evolution as reflected in the differing degrees of specialisation of the discrete neurological systems underpinning these senses in different non-human species. For example, whilst olfaction, the capacity to smell, has become relatively less important in the course of human evolution, it is a common observation that it may become more used, and useful, in people who have had long-term loss of one or more of the other four senses.

Putting ideas into practice

The scope of stimulation programs was considerably broadened by the GIO's approval of the study of coma arousal at Westmead Hospital. For the first time, it became possible for Freeman to have the support provided by a number of nurses with full-time commitment to overseeing programs to be undertaken, in collaboration with families, in the hospital. Observations made by these nurses identified very practical ways of providing less orthodox avenues for stimulation. Perhaps predictably, these related to nursing rather than medical care and so their value was not readily acknowledged by other hospital staff. As Freeman has written:

The nurses had found that the patients relaxed in a bath of warm water and that passive movement of the arms and legs was much more gentle for the patients than 'dry' work; however, our nurses were instructed (by the hospital administration) not to continue to bathe the patients. Furthermore, they were directed not to take the patients outside the airconditioned hospital into the fresh air and sunshine. We had observed that it was often in the gardens that patient awareness could be seen for the first time as the patient turned his head to look towards the sun or the surroundings.

Whilst this major expansion of resources enabled Freeman to translate his evolving ideas into practice on a scale not previously possible, it was constrained, as alluded to above, by a divergence between the goals of Freeman and those of hospital personnel. Whereas he envisaged rehabilitation as entailing an ongoing commitment to management that was not to cease *after* awakening, others considered that this event should terminate the provision of stimulation. Apart from the disagreement over when stimulation should cease, there had been some resistance within the hospital in relation to which measures could be adopted to provide stimulation. In talking with families of young patients with brain injury, Freeman usually suggested that, given appropriate conditions, improvement may be expected to continue, albeit at a decreasing rate, throughout the remainder of their lives.

This divergence in interpretation of what the project was actually to be about did not bite until some time after initiation of the preliminary feasibility study for the trial. At this stage, the numbers of 'emerged' patients began to accumulate. Whilst some of these people were admitted into existing hospital rehabilitation programs, Freeman's concerns lay especially with others who, whilst awake and aware, remained locked in. This disagreement came to a head in 1985. Freeman and his collaborators wrote to the hospital administrators spelling out their belief concerning the nature of therapy required by those patients who had emerged from coma. This letter, which warned of the disadvantage to them if this was not undertaken, contains a most succinct statement in response to the question regarding the future *after* emergence, which was posed in the title of the present chapter. Freeman wrote:

Since the initial application to the Research and Ethics Committee the feasibility project has clearly identified that environmental stimulation to the point where a patient can no longer be considered in coma does not take the patient to the point of being ready for the current rehabilitation service. Without this treatment, the gains made in bringing the person out of coma more quickly may well be lost in a treatment vacuum. The current rehabilitation service cannot cope with the intensity of therapy needed in this phase. Typically such a patient will wait in a high dependency ward until their own slow progression towards recovery gets them to the stage that the current rehabilitation service assesses that it can help them.

This divergence in aims led to the abandonment of the project at Westmead and the establishment, with GIO funding, of a freestanding facility in the Sydney suburb of Eastwood. This facility, the Brain Injury Therapy Centre (BITC), was able to admit patients who, having emerged from coma but being ineligible for rehabilitation within a hospital (because they failed to attain the prerequisites for entry into existing rehabilitation services), were likely to be abandoned. The BITC also assumed responsibility for day-care patients who, until that time, had been assisted in a facility at Baulkham Hills, supported by the GIO. The subsequent period during which the BITC operated was notable for the complete implementation of Freeman's strategies for longer-term rehabilitation.

Funding for provision of rehabilitation to patients entering the BITC was provided irrespective of their insurance status. This was not so for other institutions. The timely availability of financial compensation influenced the possible support for rehabilitation available to patient and family once the acute stage had passed. Apart from insurance status, the issue of whether, and to what extent, the patient was conscious could have a substantial impact on the size of the continuing financial support to be provided as compensation. If a patient was accepted as being in a persistent vegetative state, the extent of ongoing support that would be provided was considerably less than that which would be considered reasonable for a similar patient who, it was acknowledged, had regained some level of awareness. Essentially, the level of support in the first situation might amount to little more than very basic nursing measures. Consequently, there was a strong incentive for lawyers retained by any insurer to obtain an expert medical opinion to certify that a patient remained in a persistent vegetative state.

Recognition by the GIO that comprehensive resourcing of rehabilitation offered an opportunity to improve the outcome for brain injured people by reducing their level of dependency, and ultimately to reduce costs on the industry, led to the funding of the BITC. This incentive was reinforced by a strong humanitarian commitment on the part of the GIO staff with whom Ted Freeman interacted, and entry to the BITC was determined by the likelihood that a patient could benefit from it. As mentioned above, a patient's insurance status was irrelevant. As a result, Freeman was able for a period to provide inpatient rehabilitation in a manner that he considered optimal. Support provided by the BITC prepared residents for transition to domiciliary programs with ongoing support from the centre's staff.

Freeman has given an account of the transfer from the hospital to the BITC:

We breathed a sigh of relief when we cleared our desks, collected our documentation and equipment and parted company with Westmead Hospital. The conflict over the preceding 20 months had been emotionally demanding. The clinical nurses in the team had been extraordinarily tolerant and long-suffering for the sake of the patients and their families. The whole team transferred to St Edmund's Hospital in Eastwood. St Edmund's had been an old-fashioned cottage hospital. Facilities were limited at first and conditions difficult. The hospital consisted of a large house with rooms that had served as the wards and we accommodated our patients in these rooms. Six patients insured by the GIO were transferred with us from Westmead Hospital. We closed the Day Therapy Centre at Baulkam Hills and those patients also came to the facility at Eastwood.

Two general practitioners with an excellent reputation provided clinical care for our patients and had total control of the patients' medical treatment. If these doctors said a patient was too sick to receive therapy, it was withheld.

Another house in the grounds, once renovated, became the Therapy Centre. Until the renovation was completed we hired a large tent in which we gave the patients their therapy. This was far from ideal. It was very hot in the summer and in wet weather the grounds became waterlogged and mushy, but the staff worked with total dedication. One night, after a particularly long spell of rain, the tent finally collapsed.

A splendid team of experienced nurses now worked at the Therapy Centre. In order to cope with the different aspects of the work, the three nurses in authority were given different streams of vocation.

One nurse, with wide experience in the wards at Westmead, Bev Burrell, was the obvious choice as the acute-care nurse.

She assessed patients in acute-care hospitals when requested by the families and only when permission had been granted by the attending doctor. These patients were generally still in coma, but out of the life-threatened state. She examined them and documented their condition before writing a program, which she taught to the families. This meant that she travelled widely throughout both the city and the country areas in New South Wales and also the other States. She became very adept at diagnosing the condition of the patients and was a great help to families lost in the medical system. She frequently encountered the displeasure of the authorities at hospitals she visited [perhaps as a surrogate for Freeman].

A second sister, Robyn Sedger, took charge of the Brain Injury Therapy Centre at Eastwood. She supervised the other registered nurses (RNs) and coordinated the families and volunteers as they provided therapy.

This became a massive job as the number of patients gradually increased to twenty-three. Her very diplomatic and careful manner ensured that all patients were properly cared for and their families supported through the most difficult times. Volunteers from the Eastwood area and other parts of Sydney came in abundance. Many were mature-age people who could use their life experience to relate to the patients. Often this involved small actions like encouraging a person to move a thumb or a finger so that communication could be established with the use of a computer keyboard. Slowly, people who had minimal movement increased their muscle range, coordination and strength. These small achievements brought a sense of liberation to the patient and were applauded by the volunteers and the staff. The younger and fitter volunteers worked with patients who were 'pumping iron': pulling weights with their hands or standing on tilt tables or riding on exercise bicycles. Often there were three or four patients in a room being helped by volunteers and supervised by a member of the nursing staff.

GIO provided a heated swimming pool and each patient was given the opportunity of floating and working in the water under the care and supervision of the instructor. Those who were incontinent had body wetsuits provided and were not denied this special type of therapy. There was such camaraderie in the centre that the atmosphere of hopelessness that permeated some rehabilitation centres had no possibility of surfacing here amongst the noise, the bustle and the excitement. One of the volunteers, a sister from St Joseph's Convent, wrote about the work being done at St Edmund's:

I feel very strongly about the work done there and the quality of life we can give these patients who otherwise would be put in nursing homes. What is life about but Love, Sharing, Caring and even the smallest improvement is rejoiced in by all patients, staff, relatives, friends and us volunteers. There is life and joy here. Come see for yourselves.

A third senior sister, Yvonne Ayrey, took charge of the development and control of domiciliary rehabilitation—our third stream of intervention.

She travelled throughout the State at the request of families who had decided to take their patient home rather than put them in an institution. This move from hospital or nursing home to a patient's home demanded a great deal from the family, but our nursing sister quickly became an expert at assessing the patient and the family situation, working out possible therapy for the patient and meeting with the volunteers from the community to teach them how to provide the therapy.

These three nurses were all first rate and each gathered assistants with the same dedication, commonsense and compassion. An additional four experienced personnel—all excellent—were added to the nursing staff. With the grapevine of communication actively working, many families contacted us to see if we could help when they had been told that 'nothing further could be done' for their brain injured relative, or that 'the end of the road had been reached', or 'what you see is what you've got'.

Freeman's account of the BITC identifies the features that sharply differentiated his approach from that prevailing in the mainstream healthcare system. Care of residents was undertaken by a team of highly experienced nurses. Recruited to assist under their direction were volunteers from the community bringing a range of backgrounds, interests and skills. Apart from the quantitative difference of the BITC from conventional hospital care in the ratio of carers to residents, there was opportunity for an even more significant qualitative distinction. An example of this described above was the availability of volunteers to assist residents to use finger movements as a means of communication. The time-consuming nature of activities of this type would preclude hospital staff from committing to them. An allocation of several sessions of 'rehab' each week could not accommodate such intensive involvement.

Unlimited access of family members to patients could enhance the work of other volunteers by ensuring a sense of security from day to day. Inclusion of family members in programs also served as a preliminary to domiciliary rehabilitation, which remained the ultimate goal of the BITC. Integration of BITC activities into patient care in the home, either after a period as a resident in the BITC or as an alternative when distance precluded regular family attendance at Eastwood, was another integral feature of the Freeman approach (the example of Joe's father in undertaking a 400 km round trip each day in order to participate in activities at the BITC, while inspiring, could not realistically be copied by most families).

All of these human activities occurred within a physical location unlike that practicable in a modern hospital, where throughput of people requiring inpatient treatment for acute conditions is essential in order to achieve maximum outcomes from bed occupancy. Not only would an acute-care hospital setting for BITC programs have been an unacceptable diversion of resources from the duties of the institution but it also would be clearly less satisfactory for the participants. Accommodation in a domestic setting with daily opportunity for outside experience accorded with the aim of maximising variation in stimulation opportunity.

Taken together, the human contribution with its mix of professional and volunteer participation located in a domestic-scale physical environment, more closely resembling that with which residents would have been familiar during their life before brain injury, promoted the creation of a unique ambience. As encapsulated in the quotation from the sister from St Joseph's Convent who was one of the volunteers, the BITC 'epitomised life and joy'.

The BITC challenged

As referred to above, the work of the BITC was very adversely affected by an attack on it by the NSW Health Minister. In the immediate aftermath of the parliamentary attack on the centre there was consternation among the residents' families and the staff. Nevertheless, the activities within the centre and the two operations undertaken in the community under its auspices continued. At this time, Ted Freeman felt that he should step back from a close supervisory role in the centre, and sought an alternative administrative arrangement for it. He suspected that much of the antagonism being publicly expressed towards the centre was directed at him personally and might abate with his withdrawal from day-to-day involvement. In seeking to set up an alternative arrangement, he made a decision that he was soon to regret. His selection of a person with financial experience together with marketing skills to administer the centre was intended to reverse the decline in funding, and the ensuing curtailment of services, which followed the adverse publicity generated by the parliamentary attack.

On her appointment, the new administrator engaged major legal and accountancy firms to work for the centre. Freeman recalls watching with increasing concern over the following months, as 'there was an extraordinary securing of funds including a large loan from a financial institution'. At this time he withdrew from all clinical involvement with the BITC and resolved to retire. The situation worsened dramatically when the administrator returned from a visit to the United States with ideas for major development of the BITC. Freeman remembers by then having 'a distinct feeling of unease about her management although [he was] unsure what action to take'. His impression that the centre was losing its soul as relations between its staff and the administrator progressively deteriorated was confirmed when the entire senior nursing staff resigned.

In response to this crisis, the Australian Brain Foundation terminated its connection with its Brain Injury Division, which was then disbanded. It was replaced with a new group, designated as the Australian Brain Injury Institute, with the BITC administrator as its executive director. A finance director and a public relations manager were appointed, the former having the brief of raising $20 million. With failure to achieve this, the board became concerned. The executive director was dismissed and the overseeing body went into liquidation. The largest circulation Sydney daily tabloid devoted its front page to an investigation by police into suspicions of financial mismanagement at the BITC. Freeman remembers this period as being worse than the separation from the Westmead Hospital four years earlier.

Freeman has described the events that followed the BITC debacle:

I was convinced that I must now retire if my work was to be assessed correctly. In January 1990, a retirement dinner was arranged for me in Sydney at which Dr Malcolm Mackay spoke eloquently of the plight of people who had sustained a brain injury and the long-term effects on their families. The Board of the Brain Injury Division was then disbanded and connections with the Australian Brain Foundation were terminated. Chris Snow recorded that a new organisation had been formed to care for patients with brain injury; however, this organisation foundered after some months.

Dorothy and I discussed in detail what action we should take. It was obvious that we would have to sell our house in Sydney—a fact that was most distressing to Dorothy as she loved the cottage and its location and we had many friends in the area. We had also just completed an extension that had given me an office and shifted me from the dining room, which previously I had cluttered with my computer and books.

We put the house on the market. Fortunately, it sold quickly but as the mortgage rates at that time were 17 per cent, we only had a couple of thousand dollars after the sale. I needed an income quickly as we had several children at university and some still at school and my previous occupations on the mission in Vanuatu and as the medical superintendent at Gosford had all been relatively lowly paid compared with a private medical practice. We could have returned to the Central Coast but with our family in Sydney this was not a good option.

I was fortunate to find work at a medical centre run by an excellent practitioner, on the Northern Beaches of Sydney; but my heart still hankered to be with people with a brain injury and their families. One day the phone rang and a person greeted me with 'Hello, Ted, this is Annette on the phone. I have had a hard job finding you. Bruce and I wondered whether you would be prepared to come and see John again? We were very distressed about what happened at the Centre but no-one else seems to want to help.'

I thought about my answer quickly and said, 'Lovely to hear from you, Annette, and I would be very happy to come and see John again. Could you give me your address.' So I started again.

Word spread rapidly amongst the families who had been treated as outpatients at the BITC. Each day brought more phone calls from families of previous patients. Many families, new to me but seeking help when the established healthcare system failed them, also made contact.

Within two months I had resigned from the medical centre and found I had more than enough patients to keep me busy every day. The calls came from all around Australia, often with, 'Are you the Dr Ted Freeman who treats people with brain injury? If so, I would like you to come and see my son/ daughter, husband/wife.'

This third period of commitment to assisting people with brain injury following the closure of the BITC had not been anticipated by Freeman at the time of that closure. During it, his activities took the form of driving to family homes throughout New South Wales in order to design and supervise individual programs. In undertaking this, he combined both his original role at the BITC and that of the nursing sister responsible for the supervision of BITC domiciliary programs described above. After a period, he was awarded a Commonwealth grant, which provided a modest level of support for him to do this. Provision of any specialised nursing or paramedical care was not included in his grant.

Whilst this period superficially resembled that following his departure from Peat Island two decades earlier, it differed in the level of awareness of his methods among members of the healthcare industry. He had demonstrated what could be done and had aroused concerns in many about the inadequacies in the long-term management of brain injury. In doing this, he had also refined considerably his ideas on how a domiciliary response to rehabilitation could be implemented.

It was not long before the Freeman practice extended throughout New South Wales and into Queensland. He has provided a graphic description of his practice:

I drove an old, green 1960s Triumph 2000 car inherited from Dorothy's mother's estate and this was soon travelling widely through Sydney and beyond. Only once did it hold me up on the road out near Windsor but I treated it gently and never drove it too fast. As soon as I could, I replaced it with a second-hand 1986 Toyota Cressida with 90 000 km on the clock.

The spread of patients meant a considerable amount of travel, and I soon had the week organised in the Sydney area. Every three months I would arrange to see patients in the NSW country towns like Tamworth, Armidale, Tweed Heads and Taree, and also travelled to Queensland to see patients in Toowoomba, Maryborough, the Sunshine Coast and the Gold Coast.

In relating his financial arrangements, it is not difficult to envisage that he shared much in common with many of the families that he visited:

We had a small Franklin caravan, which Dorothy and I would load with our gear, attach to the Cressida and set out. We were on a low budget and needed to keep travel and accommodation costs to a minimum. In this way, we did not have motel costs, we could do our own cooking and did not need to eat in restaurants, although we did enjoy one meal before a log fire in Toowoomba. It was the middle of a bitter winter.

The majority of the patients were covered by Medicare, and many had exhausted their finances as they sought help to improve the person they loved. Very few could contribute any money for travel costs and I rarely asked them for it unless they appeared to be affluent. Even if they had insurance cover often there was a dispute and the insurance company would refuse to provide any finance for therapy until the legal position was resolved. In some patients it seemed the insurance company withheld resources on the basis that the patient was likely to die without any funds being expended.

When the patient survived, their medical problems often became subservient to the massive legal machinery that had to develop to bring a legal action to the court. A legal case could continue for years until a time could be fixed when the solicitors for both the plaintiff and the defendant felt the matter could go to court. Even then, a date for a court hearing could take months to obtain.

Sharing of circumstances between doctor and patient's family probably augmented the natural rapport that Ted Freeman possessed, already remarked on in the families' letters of appreciation. From his description of this period, it is likely that the Freeman family typified many of those whom they visited in terms of financial resources.

We rented a house in Sydney for one year but renting irritated me because I could never really change anything in the house or garden and I like to potter and fiddle with the gardens and houses. We decided to obtain a mortgage and buy a small two-bedroom, fibro-roofed weatherboard house on a small block of land at Mona Vale, built about 1920. It was a ramshackle place. It had old-fashioned sliding wooden windows in the front that were falling to bits and would not close properly. There was a small loungeroom, with an open fireplace, which led into the kitchen, which linked with the back verandah. The bathroom was large with a black-painted concrete floor, an

*old toilet and a shower similar to the ones that could be found in old seaside
tourist areas. The laundry was a small separate building at the rear. The
larger bedroom became my office.*

*Various people who came were concerned about our 'fall' but we could
function in it. One family member was heard to remark to another: 'Dot
and Ted have come down in the world, haven't they?' We had made home
in many countries and always felt that if we had each other and the family
we would make do.*

*When I travelled to see patients I spent a considerable amount of time
assessing them. I always explained the diagnosis, the future possibilities
and demonstrated the program of therapy to the family. As one mother told
my brother John, 'Ted was the only doctor we have ever met who seemed to
know how to examine my son'.*

The 'Freeman approach' to domiciliary rehabilitation was ideal for the patients
but it did not conform with Medicare's computerised profiles for practice.
A consultation of several hours with the family rather than with a patient
eventually came to departmental notice and led to provision of a modest level of
funding sufficient to enable Freeman's State-wide practice to continue.

*Fortunately, even though I had a higher surgical degree, I had never
registered on the specialists' lists and I could function as a general
practitioner. This meant that patients did not need to be referred by another
medical practitioner. Families could seek a consultation directly with me.*

*The downside was that while I could claim for a prolonged house call, the
Medicare payment for this was relatively small. I had to cover travel and
the costs of medical indemnity as well as computer, telephone and postage
costs. Since I had no allowance for sickness or injury, I had to insure against
these costs myself.*

*In June 1993, Senator Graham Richardson was the Federal Minister for
Health. Some people familiar with my work, through personal involvement
as volunteers with friends whose family member had suffered a severe
brain injury, made contact with Senator Richardson on an informal basis.*

At the same time, Professor Roger Rees wrote from Adelaide to Senator
Richardson in support:

Indeed it is generally estimated that approximately 5000 persons per
year, mostly male and mostly young, experience severe traumatic brain
injury largely as the result of road accidents. For large numbers of this

group there is little hope of recovery given the more traditional methods of care in nursing homes and long stay rehabilitation hospitals. This costs Australia billions of dollars per year.

Dr Freeman has attempted to provide alternatives largely through home based and community based care. He travels the country seeing families in need and promoting the idea that the acquisition of skills and improvement in lifestyle is possible for even the most profoundly damaged. There is much evidence that, as a result of Freeman's courageous and painstaking interventions, improvement for persons with brain injury has taken place.

Not every family will want to avail themselves of Freeman's ideas or of a move from hospital based care to community and home based care. Nevertheless there are substantial numbers of families who wish to undertake this home based rehabilitation program.[2]

Freeman's account of this period continued:

In response to this intervention, I was invited to meet with the Medical Services Adviser, Health Care Access Division, Department of Health, Housing and Community Services. He questioned me. 'What do you actually do?' I had taken six case studies to demonstrate the facts and, after a short interval, he said that he could help. He said that there was a Commonwealth Health Program Grant (HPG) that allows for the provision of unusual medical services. This replaces Medicare billing. Payment would be dependent on the number of people treated. The amount of the grant was not large, but it meant I could continue my work.

With hindsight, it is not difficult to see that Freeman's extensive practice of visiting patients around the State, although it had evolved in response to the loss of the BITC, had pioneered domiciliary rehabilitation and established that it was both practicable and effective. Reflecting on this period, Ted Freeman summarised his experience:

By the early 1990s I had seen a considerable number of patients in their own homes and had established programs of therapy for their families and friends and volunteers to follow. Sensory and emotional deprivation and personal space invasion had decreased and increased therapy was provided for the patients.

Families strengthened when they determined to control the care of the person they loved and not be at the whims of the health system. It has been

---

2   Roger Rees, Letter to Graham Richardson, 13 June 1993.

said that 'what oxygen is to the body, such is hope to the meaning of life',
and they developed hope. The patients and families also benefited because
travelling to hospitals for therapy was reduced and there was no more
hanging around impersonal institutions waiting for assessment or therapy.
I always went with an expectation that there would be some positives in
both the patient and the family. I was rarely disappointed.

The usual 'medical model' had failed dismally and had little relevance to
the problems of these patients and families. Most patients were not acutely
sick. They did not require medical attention every day or every week or
every month. They only needed medical intervention on an irregular basis
if they became ill.

The way forward for them was not by more medical involvement but by
education. It was the educational model that could act positively. But
medicine was like a dog with a bone: it hung on when it had no justification
to do so.

Not every patient improved, but even those patients who changed little had
a much better social life interacting with the people who loved them and
cared about them, rather than being left in limbo in a nursing home. But, of
course, I understand that not every family is in a position to take their loved
one home; circumstances dictate what can be undertaken.

In summary, in this third period, following the closure of the BITC, Freeman's
activities took the form of driving to family homes throughout New South
Wales in order to design and supervise individual programs. Whereas the
preceding period during which the BITC was operational demonstrated what
could be undertaken with a full-time team working in association with families
and volunteers, this final period established what could be achieved by families
and volunteers unsupported by such a team. The next chapter will examine in
some detail the manner in which attempts to trial Freeman's methods ultimately
disadvantaged those people whom they were intended to benefit.

Conclusion

Although the discussion of awakening of unconscious patients in the preceding
chapter emphasised the general inadequacy of the hospital system to provide
appropriate support at this stage of recovery, I suggest that the story in this
chapter of what happens *after* awakening discloses even larger gaps in available
care. Awakening is not often, as described in media accounts, a single, abrupt,
all-or-nothing incident in which someone who has been unconscious for six

months suddenly wakes up, jumps out of bed and asks for directions to the dining room. Frequently, the first signs of awakening may be quite transient, indeed sufficiently so that their very occurrence is questioned.

Once the person is consistently awake, she or he is likely to have considerable, often gross, limitations to what can actually be done. Frequently, these limitations will disqualify the person from graduation into the institutional rehabilitation program or, if entry is achieved, will so retard progress that the person is dropped from that program. In either case, a patient may transit from acute care to limbo.

Freeman's aim was to develop an alternative placement option, which provided a form of slow-stream rehabilitation applicable to patients who had regained consciousness, but not much more. Rather than the regular rehabilitation schedule, which would be beyond the endurance capacity of these people, or the hour per week token therapy available in an aged-care situation, the aim was to have intensive person-to-person programs, specific to the individual patient and reinforced by their conduct within familiar, small-scale surroundings.

To accomplish such an alternative care option, the GIO funded a day care centre initially and then a residential facility, the BITC. The BITC was envisaged as a placement from which patients could transfer into domiciliary rehabilitation when their progress and the availability of adequate physical facilities and carers in the home had been assured. There was to be continuity between the BITC and home with as much family input as possible into a BITC-based program followed by ongoing home visits by familiar BITC staff. In both locations, BITC and home, participation by teams of volunteers in each patient's rehabilitation program was envisaged.

As events transpired, the BITC operated for a limited period of little more than three years, which was a crushing disappointment to all involved—residents, families, staff and volunteers. On a more positive note, the centre showed what could be achieved, although, with its closure, it became necessary to undertake domiciliary rehabilitation at a much earlier stage of recovery and without the nursing support provided by the centre. This earlier transition is likely to have made the domiciliary option unavailable to families who did not have the resources required.

The success of the BITC, apart from demonstrating what *could* be done, simultaneously showed why it *could not* be done in a hospital setting. The feasibility of maintaining long-term placements and of providing a staff to carer ratio of one-to-one would be ruled out, both on logistic and economic grounds. The long-term daily entry of large numbers of volunteers into wards would present considerable problems.

The solution to these impediments to rehabilitation in a conventional institutional setting arose from necessity as much as from advanced planning. That solution amounted to de-medicalisation of the rehabilitation process. Unfortunately, recognition that any decent concept of 'distributive equity' would entail a transfer of some portion of the funding saved in the institutional setting to support the domiciliary alternative, so making this more widely available throughout the community, has yet to occur.

6. Trials and tribulations

Reference has been made in the preceding chapter to the period during which Ted Freeman had an association with the Westmead Hospital as chief investigator in a research project into severe brain injury. This association was a consequence of the award of a substantial financial grant from the NSW Government Insurance Office (GIO) intended to test his ideas for procedures to facilitate awakening patients from coma after brain injury and their subsequent rehabilitation. Freeman's association with the hospital and its receipt of the GIO grant were both terminated abruptly during the course of preparing for a clinical trial.

This chapter has two discrete parts. In the first, the story of that clinical trial and its failure to progress beyond the feasibility study is told. In the course of its telling, several issues that loomed large during this trial, but which also raise important general questions, will be identified. When the story of the trial is complete, attention is directed to these more general questions about clinical trials, which events at Westmead raise.

It should be recognised in the planning stage that double-blind randomised control trials of procedures, the outcome of which may be dependent on interpersonal relationships between research subjects and those responsible for undertaking procedures with them, may be impossible to implement. The absence from the literature of trials of coma arousal procedures that meet all the 'control' criteria may reflect this. Career implications for researchers may exist in any trial and the utmost care should be taken to anticipate them and to ensure that research aspirations do not displace clinical obligations, especially in the case of very vulnerable research subjects. Whether allocation of patient-subjects to 'non-treatment' control groups should have been considered ethically acceptable late in the twentieth century, and an associated question—namely, whether it is permissible to impose foreseeable risks on a *control* group—are considered.

Background to the 'Westmead experience'

Prior to his association with Westmead Hospital, Freeman had been receiving support from the GIO to investigate the possible use of stimulation in order to facilitate the emergence of people with brain injuries from coma and then to continue their rehabilitation. In 1983, earlier discussion about a possible trial led to the development of a protocol for it. Whilst the hospital administration was receptive to accepting the funding to undertake the study, Freeman sensed possible difficulties. He attributed these to widespread adherence to the opinion prevalent among Australian rehabilitation practitioners that sensory input to comatose patients should be minimised. This opinion held not only that it was not helpful, but also that it might disadvantage a patient. Freeman recalled:

> *Stimulation of the person in coma was diametrically opposed to the thinking prevailing at that time with regard to the treatment of brain injury, but it was obvious to me that providing an input to the comatose patient through vision, hearing and touch, as long as it was kept within normal sensations, could not be dangerous.*

Reinforcing opposition to the use of stimulation, concerns existed among many professionals about allowing (non-professional) family members to provide that stimulation. As will be apparent from earlier chapters, especially the patients' stories, Freeman's experiences had convinced him that assisting and/or detecting returning consciousness could be facilitated with assistance from family members at the earliest possible stage. He found that this was not generally accepted:

> *The head of a department at one hospital was quoted as saying, 'You might as well hang a bunch of bananas at the end of the bed. It would have the same effect as this coma arousal!' I thought that remark was hardly a scientific approach to the imperative of finding new ways to solve a major problem!*

The 'banana' remedy proved not to be an isolated incident, as Freeman soon realised. Doctors who would have clinical responsibility for patients admitted to the trial were frequently unwilling to monitor their progress on a regular basis. Some hospital staff expressed anxiety that the trial would attract premature and unwelcome media attention. Access to patients was not always forthcoming. Notwithstanding these impediments, a financial solution, even if only temporary, was at hand. Acceptance by the hospital of the study was settled when the GIO offered to donate $20 000, which the hospital needed for the purchase of equipment unrelated to the study.

Setting up the feasibility study

By the end of 1983, the protocol had been scrutinised and passed by the Ethics and Research Committee of the Westmead Hospital and the GIO decided to fund a feasibility study on coma arousal at the hospital as a preliminary to a full-scale exercise. Freeman anticipated some difficulties in mounting the trial because of the number of different hospital departments whose cooperation would be essential. While the research protocol for administration of therapy to patients was thorough, there were no clear, existing guidelines outlining the method by which the research could be integrated with the normal functioning of the hospital. Apart from difficulties peculiar to the specific trial, there were probably some general obstacles that may have arisen with any large trial in a hospital unaccustomed to trials. Freeman recalls that little effort was made within the hospital to integrate the trial requirements into a number of different departments.

The feasibility study was intended to be the prelude for a full-scale investigation of Freeman's procedures, provided it appeared to support his contention that there were obvious gains in the use of coma arousal. He anticipated some management difficulties:

> *Whilst arousal procedures had previously been implemented intuitively and informally by some families in the hospital or the patient's home by laypersons (not hospital employees), it was considered that they could potentially be disruptive for the care of patients, both those in the study and others coincidentally located close to them.*

The aims of the feasibility study were

1. to determine if coma arousal could be carried out in the wards of a general hospital

2. to find out if the relatives of patients with brain injury could provide the arousal program

3. to determine whether, on the basis of probability, there was some advantage to be gained for the patients.

Once the go-ahead for the study had been obtained, it was necessary to recruit the best available personnel to undertake the dual function of supervising the programs and maintaining good rapport with the ward staff. Freeman explained the basis for his decision as follows:

> *It was necessary to select a team leader. The choice was a nurse, physiotherapist, occupational therapist or social worker. I chose a nurse because, in my experience, the nurse is multi-skilled while the other disciplines tend to specialise in one area. The nursing professionals are generally competent when dealing with a mess. If the patient vomits or defecates or passes urine, the nurse is not fazed but will clean the patient and continue with the work. The other professionals will call for a nurse to remedy the situation. I also thought that it was important for the therapist to be able to touch the patient and this excluded a social worker.*

In the event, he appointed a nurse with experience of neurosurgery wards who was highly recommended by the hospital director of nursing. She was a very practical nurse, with a great capacity for hard work, the ability to understand the objectives of the research, and to apply the research in a practical working situation. She established excellent rapport with relatives. Having once made up her mind, she was committed to her way of carrying out the therapy unless there were good reasons to change. This determination on her part ensured a standard of high quality for both the patients and the families.

Freeman was soon to become aware of the difficulties that were likely to arise when management that had empirically been found to benefit a particular group of patients was to be submitted to the scientific requirements of a randomised trial. Perhaps even sooner, he encountered the demarcations underlying the operation of any large hospital. He was aware of the potential for rivalry between different professional disciplines and for territorial disputes within hospitals. His choice of a nurse triggered such a dispute, with at least one of the occupational therapists vowing to get one of his own as team leader.

An issue that is of primary importance in consideration of any clinical trial is that of possible harm to the patient. The clinical trial at Westmead was most unusual in that it was necessary to consider not only risks of harm to participating patients but also the risks of adverse effects on their (equally participating) families. The possibility that families might be adversely affected by participation in a trial was one of which Freeman was well aware.

Some observations made at an early stage during the feasibility study, by two of the social workers in the research team, were relevant to assessing this risk. These observations concerned the adverse effects, already triggered by the event of the brain injury per se, on family members, antedating entry into the trial. Before any attempt to identify adverse consequences of participation in the trial could be undertaken, it was necessary to assess the residual impact of the event of the brain injury itself. Two social workers in the team evaluated the attitudes of families who were about to enter the trial. These were invariably heavily influenced by the event that had occasioned the brain injury to their family member. The social workers in the coma arousal team reported:

> This event was often reported as the most tragic event in their lives. There were deep fears for their relative's survival, and for survival in what state; guilt for wondering whether their relative would be better off dead than the possibility of remaining in the vegetative state; guilt about their inability to stop the accident happening—'If only I had not let her go out with them'; bargaining—'Why not me, I've lived longer?'; disbelief, shock, numbness; bewilderment at a hospital and intensive care unit; fear and anger; days merging into one; terror when the phone rings at night; insomnia.

Commenting upon the ability of family members to cope with, and adjust to, the catastrophe that had befallen their family member, Freeman reflected:

Over the years I have found that generally the women in the family cope better than the men when their relative is in the early stages of brain injury. Men, especially those who have been in positions where they are required to take charge of situations, often suffer the typical stress reaction of 'fight or flight' because they suddenly feel powerless in the face of this terrible event that has befallen their family.

The practicality of conducting a trial in hospital wards without disrupting normal operations was affirmed as early as May 1984 by the Director of Nursing, who wrote to Freeman in the following terms:

I wish to advise, following discussions with the nursing staff, that the Coma Arousal Study has caused no disruption to the ward involved. The presence of family members has not interfered in any way with the nursing care and the only effect the study has had on the nursing staff has been advantageous. All of the staff are extremely interested in the program and the favourable responses to therapy from the patient.

By September 1984, another potential adverse consequence for participating families appeared not to be a cause for concern. The social workers who had previously evaluated the residual impact on families of the injury to the patients reported:

Families were unanimous that the program had been positive for them. The families believed the coma arousal team gave help to the patient as well as understanding to the families of the changes as the patient progressed. These things gave a sense of control. It took away their feelings of isolation and hopelessness and demystified the medical system. It removed many of their misconceptions and fears and unified the family with a common purpose and approach. The only criticism of the program was that it should have started earlier.

On the basis of the social workers' report, and of his personal observations, Freeman concluded that families could successfully participate in a trial:

The relatives acknowledged that sharing information with members of other families was beneficial because, knowing what it was like to be in this terrible predicament, they became a source of mutual support for each other, especially as they found it difficult to talk to the neurosurgeons, all of whom appeared to be too busy after the first week. This was understandable as the neurosurgeons were involved in life-saving surgery and were constantly in demand for the next acute admissions.

This was positive news, implying not only that families were unlikely to be adversely affected by their involvement in a program, but also that they gained encouragement from it. Another finding—namely, that families provided mutual support to each other—foreshadowed complications for implementing a randomised control trial. It hardly required penetrating insight to appreciate that daily communication between families would render it both morally and humanely indefensible to allow some families (in the 'experimental'—that is, active—group) to participate in 'hands-on' involvement for their family members whilst others (the 'control', passive, group) were precluded from doing so.

By October 1984, it was possible to summarise some of the findings with the 12 patients in the feasibility study. One had died, three were at home, four were ready to go to the rehabilitation department, three were still on the program, one of whom was out of coma, and one other patient had not responded and had been taken off the program.

Alongside this positive preliminary finding, the feasibility study had exposed, as such studies are intended to do, some major potential complications inherent in upgrading to a full-scale trial. Freeman summarised these as:

1. There was no clinical document in use to assess the small but important changes in the early stages as the person aroused from coma.

2. Drugs were sometimes used excessively or for too long. While necessary in the acute stage of treatment, many were given in high doses for weeks and months. Many of these drugs were highly sedative—enough to prevent the patient from waking.

3. Tubes were left in the nose and into the trachea far longer than necessary.

Freeman regarded this as totally unacceptable and a violation of the intimate personal space of the patient. He recalled:

The team was dismayed to find patients with their arms tied to the armrests on the chairs because they 'tried to pull their tubes out'. If the patient tried to pull out the tubes, their body language implied that it was time to check if the tubes could be removed safely.

4. The physiotherapists sometimes applied plasters (plaster of Paris) similar to those that are used to treat people with broken bones. This was done in an attempt to prevent muscle contraction; but the problem of muscle contraction following a brain injury was totally different from that of broken bones and required a totally different method of treatment. The team wanted to provide a dynamic approach to the restoration of body function, but the plasters prevented the application of stimulation to the skin by touch or vibration or pressure or the application of ice. They also prevented any attempts to rotate, extend or flex the arm or leg through its normal range of movements.

Mounting a trial

Responding to the results of the feasibility study early in 1985, the GIO decided to offer funding for a more extensive study. This was to be a full-scale prospective study running over three years. GIO offered to provide $1 million to Westmead and $500 000 for development of a research protocol by the Commonwealth Institutes of Health in the University of Sydney. In the GIO letter offering this funding, it was specified that the money was to be used to establish a Coma Arousal Unit in Westmead Hospital, as described by Dr Freeman, in which treatment was to be provided under his supervision. GIO funds went directly to the finance section of the Westmead Hospital. Freeman was not involved in their disbursement.

The unit envisaged would be the first of its kind in a major Australian teaching hospital. There were some specialised units overseas, such as the Royal Hospital for Neurodisability in London, specifically concerned with coma arousal, but these were not located within general teaching hospitals. The GIO expressed the hope that the new unit would lead the way to a dynamic approach to the management of severe brain injury. The hospital accepted the GIO offer in February 1985, indicating that it was seeking to provide optimal physical facilities for the project within the constraints of resources available. The awarding of the grant was announced in the NSW Parliament and attracted considerable media attention.

Two weeks after the announcement of the grant, Freeman was speaking with an American friend, who remarked, somewhat prophetically, 'Ted, with money like that, your problems are now about to begin. You will have a battle to keep the research under your control.' True to forecast, the arrangement was to become completely unworkable before the end of the year.

The first problem to arise concerned the proposed structure of the trial. Epidemiological input from the School of Public Health at the university favoured a double-blind randomised control trial as the most rigorous design. In this type of trial, subjects who have 'matched' medical conditions are randomly allocated to one of two treatment groups. One group will receive the treatment regimen that the trial is intended to test. The other receives the alternative (control) treatment with which it is to be compared. In a double-blind trial, neither the medical personnel responsible for treatment of the two groups nor others responsible for assessing the results should be aware of which group any patient is in.

Freeman expressed ethical concerns. The allocation of some patients to a control group, which meant in practice 'no treatment', was unacceptable to him. He expressed a preference for a trial in which each patient acted as his/her own control. He considered that

> [w]here the patient outcome is acknowledged internationally to be disastrous, the withholding of such a non-invasive, atraumatic, non-surgical treatment was unwarranted. Today it is recognised that at times the epidemiological demands may jeopardise the optimum treatment of the patient, in which case most clinicians see the patient's treatment as taking absolute priority.

Two other envisaged features of the trial were at odds with Freeman's philosophy. How was the management of people who had 'emerged', consistently or intermittently, albeit remaining 'locked in' and unable to communicate, to be accommodated within any trial? How sound, ethically and scientifically, was the termination of stimulation procedures for the 'experimental' group after 10 weeks, irrespective of the condition of the subject at that time, in order to create a 'clean' universal cut-off point for data analysis? In relation to the second question, Freeman was informed by a hospital administrator in April 1985 that:

> One major problem seems to be in defining when the patient comes out of coma and hence an endpoint to the need of coma arousal. My impression is that you now wish to continue a treatment program beyond the point of arousal from coma and into the rehabilitation phase of patient care. This is outside the scope of your present research proposal and is being seen to impinge on the responsibilities of other hospital staff.

Apparently, this difficulty was not directly concerned with requirements imposed by the trial but, rather, with the territorial instincts that are a common feature of healthcare communities. Continuation of a program was considered to trespass on the responsibilities of the hospital's rehabilitation practitioners. While, most importantly, premature termination could cut across patients' opportunities for later improvement, it could also preclude chances of the trial actually discovering something. The emerging complications were considered by hospital personnel, who then contacted Freeman:

> It is clear that the program is beset with a number of problems and that it will not be possible to enter the next stage of the study, the controlled clinical trial, until these have been resolved. Much of our present problem results from the fact that the treatment conducted in

the feasibility study extended beyond your original brief. What was originally presented as coma arousal therapy has extended to prolonged intensive rehabilitation.

It was recorded above that a study undertaken by social workers in the 'coma arousal' team as part of the feasibility study had emphasised the beneficial manner in which patients' families interacted with each other to provide mutual support. This interaction, however, was identified in a report to the hospital's Research and Ethics Committee as a hazard to the research. This report warned that such interaction

> would lead to a serious contamination of the treatment and control groups because of the fact that relatives often spend long times in the hospital in a highly emotional state … There is considerable interchange between the different sets of relatives while they are waiting at this hospital and given the situation and the fact that they are seeking information about possibilities of improvement from any source possible, it is impossible to stop leakage of the treatment procedures.

'Contamination' was an unfortunate choice of terms, perhaps unintentionally disclosing where the balance between subject welfare and research needs lay. It indicated quite unequivocally where the priorities of the author(s) of the report to the Research and Ethics Committee lay. A further unfortunate, albeit revealing, choice of vocabulary appeared in correspondence, in this instance, from hospital personnel to the university. A senior doctor wrote, on 16 May 1985, concerning 'the firm opinion that this study cannot be allowed to proceed unless both control and treated patients are from Westmead Hospital'.

If this were not done, he was of the view that 'no self respecting editor [of a journal] would allow a study with such a basic design fault to be published'.

This opinion inevitably raises the issue of for *whose* benefit the trial was to be undertaken. Potential conflict between the personal interests of the participating subjects (that is, patients) and the career aspirations of the researchers may arise in any study and should, it seems reasonable to argue, invariably be resolved in favour of the former. Freeman's account of the media presentation of the awarding of the GIO grant suggested that considerable kudos was attached to the receipt of such a large grant on the part of both recipient institutions.

As a means of avoiding 'contamination' because of contact between families, it was suggested by some of the Westmead practitioners that 'control' (passive) patients be at that hospital while the trial (active) group should be located at Parramatta Hospital. Another suggested approach intended to assist with undertaking the trial entailed the replacement of the control group with data drawn from an existing source, such as the US National Coma Data Bank.

Accompanying this alternative was a proposal to replace family members with professional therapists whose input could be more readily standardised, perhaps assisting the process of outcome measurement. This proposal indicated a failure to grasp the manner in which a family's intimate knowledge of their patient could equip its ability to tailor procedures to provide the best chances of success for that individual. This is clearly a situation in which one size does not fit all. Not unexpectedly, Freeman disagreed forcefully with the proposal to use professional therapists. As he argued:

> *It was my belief that the relatives had so much to offer the patient because they knew the patient intimately and were highly motivated to do the work. 'No-one is more motivated than me to get my child better,' exclaimed one father when I asked him if the demands of the therapy on him were too great.*

Freeman's intuitive belief that family participation in programs is highly desirable receives considerable support from the recent electrical studies of brain function described in Chapter 4. For instance, these studies demonstrated that, when an investigator spoke about people and topics with personal relevance to the unconscious patient, unique electrical responses could be detected.

Reinforcing the hospital's arguments that family participation introduced risks of 'contamination' and of variability in the way in which different families implemented stimulation procedures, it was also contended that prolonged involvement could have adverse effects on family members. Similar arguments suggesting that stimulation procedures risked introducing 'false hope' were regularly raised, independently of the trial, by those critical of Freeman's approach. This was at odds with the observations of the social workers in the team noted above, but in response to the objection Freeman suggested to the hospital management that an independent examination of the effects on families of participation in arousal programs should be undertaken. His request did not receive any response in the rapidly deteriorating interactions with hospital authorities.

Whereas Westmead was unresponsive to Freeman's suggestion of examination of the possible effects of the trial on families, in 1986, after the project at Westmead had been discontinued, the GIO proceeded to fund an independent study by the Unit for Rehabilitation Studies at Macquarie University.[1] A few extracts from the resulting report are provided below. They represent an assessment, from the perspective of families, that was consistent with the thrust of the small questionnaire undertaken by Freeman (mentioned in Chapter 3) and of the descriptions, noted above, of the project's social workers.

---

1 Cecilia Gray, Tony J. Koop & Trevor Parmenter (1986) *Coma Care Family Survey*. Report commissioned by the Government Insurance Office of New South Wales.

One conclusion contained in the Macquarie unit's report in relation to the participating families was: 'They felt that the Coma Care staff explained fully the nature of this experimental program to them giving them no false hopes but a great deal of support, encouragement and understanding.'

The Macquarie researchers considered that participation had brought positive psychological benefits for families. They reported:

> The involvement in the Coma Arousal Program and thus contributing to the care of the patient, in the vast majority of cases, helped to relieve many of the feelings of frustration and of helplessness experienced by close relatives and friends.

Close involvement of families in programs was seen as assisting them to cope: 'This provided emotional support mitigating in part the destructive effects the patient's accident has upon their lives.' Perhaps the most revealing indication of families' attitudes towards participation in a program was elicited in response to the researchers' questioning about whether they would recommend participation to other families. They commented in the report on the response to this question as follows:

> The fact that 97% of respondents answered 'yes' to the question of whether they would advise other people to be involved in a program such as this one seems to indicate that not only was it deemed worth it for the patient but also for themselves (3% didn't respond to the question).

Of 32 respondents who were asked whether they felt like withdrawing from the program, all but one answered 'no' or, more emphatically, 'never'. All respondents to the question of whether the Coma Care Team was a support answered emphatically in the affirmative: 'Extremely supportive. He wasn't just a patient, he was an identity.'

Although the primary purpose of the survey was to assess the impact of the program's staff on families, responses provided a wider perspective. One conclusion drawn in the report was:

> Overall there was a fairly even mixture of positive and negative reactions by respondents to hospital staff, nursing staff, physiotherapists, occupational therapists, social workers and the doctors in intensive care. However, while there was unanimous agreement about the excellent quality of the Coma Care staff's treatment and support, the vast majority reported negative reactions to and relationships with neurosurgeons.

By August 1985, an approach from a senior hospital administrator to the GIO sought to retain the funding for the project while effectively sidelining

Ted Freeman from the research. This communication asserted in support of continuing the trial in this way that '[n]o-one has yet put coma arousal to the test and it should be done before demand rises to such an extent that it will be impossible to get patients in a "no treatment" condition'.

In another unfortunate, but revealing, choice of vocabulary, the writer equated the 'control' group with a 'no treatment' one. Concern was also expressed in this letter that media attention might increase demand for entry to the 'treatment' group.

A report to the GIO Board on 30 September 1985 from Kevin Beckton, the GIO person responsible for oversight of the trial, recommended that the funding be removed from the hospital. Beckton, who had by this time been closely involved with the aims of the trial from its earliest stage, supported his recommendation on two principal grounds. He regarded the hospital's proposal to remove Freeman from direct involvement as completely unacceptable. Second, he did not accept the hospital management's change in attitude to limit the trial duration to 10 weeks:

> [T]here is no doubt that the recommended duration of therapy will be 10 weeks or thereabouts, as this is the item upon which the differences of opinion most clearly have manifested themselves. Both Freeman and I agree ten weeks was inadequate and that the greatest improvements occurred after this period. I draw your attention to the fact that the proposal contained in the letter from Westmead Administration of 21st August 1985 does not attack the continuation of the scheme on the basis of harm to the patient but suggests relatives are at risk. As most of the patients have been obtained from the human scrap heap any change is probably an improvement.

The account of the preparations for the study does not mention the process that was envisaged in gaining informed consent for participation in the double-blind randomised control trial. Clearly, consent would necessarily have to be obtained from families as representatives of the patients. Equally clearly, this process would necessitate the provision to the families of an information document for a study that was to be undertaken under the auspices of two institutions of high standing in the Sydney community. An essential part of such an information sheet for a control trial would be the disclosure that only half of the patients were to be entered in a 'Freeman program'. Given that all of the patients had entered the study *because of* the regard in which they held the man and his philosophy, it beggars credulity to anticipate that *any* of the families would have opted to enter such a lottery had they been adequately informed.

Consistent with the commitment of those on Freeman's team to assisting the patients with whom they would be working, they regarded withholding of the trial therapy from any patient as unthinkable. On the other hand, the hospital clinicians envisaged having a concurrent control group. The information sheet for families of potential participants was prepared by the team and did not include any mention of a control or non-treatment group.

Apart from the unacceptability of a trial in which their family member had a 50 per cent chance of missing out on attempts at arousal (that is, the 'random' aspect of the trial), the concept of the trial being 'double blind' should have been perceived from the beginning to be entirely fatuous. An essential component of double blinding is that *neither* the doctors responsible for supervising the treatment modality under test and its control *nor* those (others) responsible for measuring the responses of the two groups should be aware of which patients were in which group. Whilst this double-blinding requirement may be readily achievable when the trial sets out to compare two pharmaceutical preparations, it becomes a nonsense to claim that the supervising doctors can remain blinded when the experimental group is to receive intensive stimulation. Supervising doctors may be suitably blinded when each group is to receive an unmarked pill, but not when a team of therapists is hovering in the background.

With hindsight, it appears almost inevitable that the Westmead trial would encounter major obstacles. There was hostility towards Freeman's ideas, and perhaps towards him personally, from some of the hospital's medical staff. There was apparently dissension within the hospital over which professional specialties should be responsible for trial conduct, and this disagreement intruded into its planning. The substantial financial support, which may have been larger than any research funding that the hospital administration had been required to manage to that time, could have fuelled some of these difficulties inherent in the trial. Leaving 'Westmead-specific' issues to the side for the moment, it is worth considering, at the distance of a quarter-century, some of the innate difficulties in clinical trials, in any location, which the coma arousal trial exemplified.

Clinical trials: Ethical considerations

The Cochrane Collaboration is an organisation established to evaluate clinical trials of drugs and treatment procedures. Its goal is to facilitate the introduction and retention in practice of treatments the scientific basis for which has been validated in the course of clinical trials. It does not undertake trials itself but conducts comprehensive searches of medical databases to assess the scientific and statistical values of published results and then to collate those which attain the required standard and to subject the aggregated data from the acceptable trials to further analysis.

In 2009, the Cochrane Library published a review entitled *Sensory Stimulation for Brain Injured Individuals in Coma or Vegetative State.*[2] The authors identified 25 published articles on this subject, but only three of these satisfied the Cochrane criteria of being randomised, double-blind trials. The assessors expressed considerable reservations even about these three. When compared with 'standard' double-blind randomised trials of new drugs, they did not measure up well.

It has always been a requirement that the information provided to people who are considering entry to a clinical trial clearly indicates that they may not personally benefit from participation. The primary goal of a clinical trial has historically been to establish whether the new treatment that is to be examined is superior to existing options and, consequently, the envisaged beneficiaries will be *other* people affected by the condition for which the new treatment is a potential remedy. More recently, research ethics committees have been required to consider trials the declared aim of which has not been to demonstrate *superiority* but only to establish *non-inferiority* of the new therapy when compared with existing ones. Committees are increasingly required to distinguish genuine trials from marketing exercises.

The largest trials are generally concerned with testing the efficacy of a pharmacological agent and hence the pharmaceutical industry is numerically by far the largest sponsor of trials. This has now developed to the extent where double-blind randomised control trials have become a major income-generating industry in themselves, with their sponsoring corporations being the major beneficiaries.

A 2011 Australian Government publication was titled *Clinically Competitive*: *Boosting the Business of Clinical Trials in Australia.* At its launch, the Ministers for Health and Ageing and for Innovation, Industry, Science and Research were quite explicit in emphasising the commercial benefits of trials for participating institutions: 'It is an industry that brings hundreds of millions of dollars annually into Australia's health system.'[3] Subjects participating in a trial are the heroes. Apart from potential benefits for society at large, the major beneficiaries may include the manufacturers of tested products and the medical personnel

---

2   Francesco F. L. Lombardi, Mariangela Taricco, Antonio de Tanti, Elena Talaro & Alessandro Liberari (2009) *Sensory Stimulation for Brain Injured Individuals in Coma or Vegetative State (Review)*. The Cochrane Collaboration. John Wiley & Sons Ltd, London.
3   Clinical Trials Action Group Report (2011) *Clinically Competitive: Boosting the Business of Clinical trials in Australia*. Ministers' foreword. Australian Government Publishing Office, Canberra.

undertaking the trial for the manufacturers. Seen in this light, the opportunity to participate in the randomised control trial of coma arousal may be considered as less of a notable win for comatose patients than for those professionals conducting the trial.

Potential exists for any trial to prejudice the clinical care of an individual patient. In designing any trial, this risk should be identified and then minimised. A survey of 500 Australian physicians and paediatricians published in 2005 concluded that '[r]elationships with patients were valued over research accomplishments and most felt that their patients' right to select treatment took precedence over advancing knowledge'.[4] It was inferred that the doctors surveyed were generally clinician oriented rather than research oriented. Judging from the conditions that were introduced into the proposed trial during the preliminary discussions, the balance between the entitlements of the comatose Westmead group as *patients* and their liabilities as *research subjects* does not appear to have been a major consideration in planning for application of the substantial GIO grant.

Whilst the issue of striking a fair balance between the interests of patients and subjects has not always been thoroughly considered, it is interesting to observe current developments in trials of new drugs. An array of the highest-profile US oncologists has divided in arguing about this balance as it relates to trialling PLX 4032, a new agent that appears to offer the possibility of significant improvement in the control of disseminated melanoma tumours. Whilst this new agent is currently the subject of a nationwide random controlled trial, many clinicians have asserted that patients who have been 'randomised' to serve as controls and consequently denied treatment with it should have access to the drug. The counterargument runs: 'Without the hard proof the trials can provide, doctors are left to prescribe unsubstantiated hope—and an overstretched health service is left to pay for it.'[5]

The common feature of the 'Westmead' trial and the PLX 4032 one is the dubious ethical acceptability of exclusion of participants in the control group from treatment that may potentially be beneficial for them. When a trial is intended to establish whether a new treatment is superior to an established procedure for which some level of efficacy has already been demonstrated, this concern about exclusion can be much less than is the case in a situation in which the control is, realistically, 'no treatment' or patently futile treatment. When an

---

4   Patrina H. Y. Caldwell, Jonathan C. Craig & Phyllis N. Butow (2005) Barriers to Australian physicians' and paediatricians' involvement in randomised control trials. *Medical Journal of Australia, 182*, 59.
5   Amy Hermon (2010) New drugs stir debate on basic rules of clinical trials. *The New York Times*, 19 September.

established treatment offering some benefit is available, the ethical concern may relate more to any possibility of adverse effects of the new treatment on subjects randomised to the experimental group.

Reverting to the 1985 trial of coma arousal therapy, a number of other issues deserve specific consideration. The assumption, implicit in any comparative trial, that each of the subjects randomised between the two groups has an equivalent pathology, remains highly questionable. Clinical similarity between two patients each of whom has sustained a brain injury can certainly not be presumed automatically to equate with identicality of structural damage.

To illustrate the nature of 'treatment' on offer to the control group, it will suffice to direct attention to the description of patient management at Weemala in an earlier chapter. Trials in which treatment is withheld from, or not available to, the control group have a disreputable history. Examples of withholding treatment that was considered to have some value in order to observe the consequences have attained permanence in the bioethical literature. Such examples include the withholding of the (admittedly imperfect) treatment then available from patients with primary-stage syphilis in Tuskegee, USA, and of minor prophylactic surgery from women with early stage cervical cancer in Auckland.[6]

The locating of a mid-1990s trial of a putatively improved treatment for neonatal AIDS in a Third-World location in which the available treatment was nil attracted much opprobrium (it was not permissible to mount such a trial capable of providing a statistically satisfactory outcome in developed nations where affordable, effective treatment was available).

Perhaps rather simplistically, the issue of whether the Westmead control group was a non-treatment group raises the question of what is treatment? In a rather revealing comment, a letter to the GIO from the epidemiologist participating in the trial (who, it was proposed, would replace Freeman as chief investigator), which sought to preserve the funding, minus Freeman, described the 'control' group as the 'no treatment group'.

One communication from the epidemiologist pressed the case for inclusion of the 'no treatment' group on the basis that media publicity about 'coma arousal' could make it impossible in the future to recruit starters for a trial in which 50 per cent of patients would effectively remain untreated. This might be read as an expedient call to undertake a trial before the provision of adequate information to participating families about what was involved would, quite reasonably, inhibit recruitment. Whilst one could acknowledge that this may have been

---

6   Phillida Bunkle (1988) *Second Opinion: The Politics of Women's Health in New Zealand*. Oxford University Press, Auckland.

epidemiologically sound, it would be difficult to provide the same unqualified reassurance about its ethical soundness. A 'worst case' interpretation could read this concern as acknowledging that ignorance of the details, among those giving consent for entry of patients into the trial, was a prerequisite.

Media coverage of any medical issue frequently tends to go 'over the top', and the perceptions of those responsible for making decisions about entry into a trial may have been distorted as a result. On the other hand, the decision-makers considering entry of a relative into any trial are entitled to be fully informed about every aspect of that trial which could affect their decision. As a minimum requirement, some reasonable attempt to balance epidemiological and ethical imperatives should have been undertaken.

Historically, the provision of basic nursing care with the administration of food and water would not generally have been designated as 'treatment'. In the past two decades, however, considerable efforts have been made to reclassify the administration of food and water to patients in prolonged coma as 'treatment', with the explicit intent of thereby reclassifying it as something that could be withheld. Advocates of this interpretation have included the US President's Commission. A 1983 paper from this august group deemed the expression 'life-sustaining treatment' as extending from the use of ventilators to 'home physical therapy, nursing support for activities of daily living and special feeding procedures'.[7] The acknowledged purpose of this new classification was to achieve legal sanction for the withdrawal of hydration and nutrition.

Clinical trials of new therapies have two main roles. Almost all attention has so far been directed to establishing efficacy of a new therapy. The second role— probably more important—is that of confirming the safety of the new treatment. It is difficult to postulate that coma arousal procedures as espoused by Freeman would be dangerous for the patient and the absence from the scientific literature of research reports of harm to patients supports this conclusion. Nevertheless, it was claimed at the time that families of patients might be psychologically harmed, a suggestion which the Macquarie University study, described above, effectively refuted.

In the absence of any documented evidence of harm to comatose individuals from heightened contact with family members, it seems equally unlikely that comatose patients would be harmed by increased family contact. In short, the risk of harm consequent upon receiving the 'experimental' protocol appears to have been nil.

---

7   President's Commission for the Study of Ethical Problems in Medicine and Biomedical and Behavioural Research (1983) *Deciding to Forgo Life-sustaining Treatment: A Report on the Ethical, Medical and Legal Issues in Treatment Decisions*. Government Printing Office, Washington, DC.

In describing the recent dispute over the US randomised control trial of melanoma therapy, the very large costs to the healthcare system of allowing widespread use of PLX 4032 as an unproven drug were cited. In the case of coma arousal therapy, it is difficult to foresee any significant new impositions on the healthcare budget if the procedure of coma arousal, as practised by families, became widespread, as the labour input would be voluntary. While this should effectively disable arguments against considering the introduction of stimulation procedures into coma arousal and ongoing rehabilitation on the grounds of imposing additional costs on 'the system', it certainly should not be taken as excusing that system from acknowledging voluntary support by reasonable budgetary compensation.

Whilst the healthcare budget is spared if a family opts for domiciliary rehabilitation, this will invariably be at the expense of the family budget. The patient stories recounted above include instances in which the primary carer was a wife, a husband, a mother or a father. Frequently, both of the last two were heavily committed. Apart from the current income forgone, the future re-employment prospects of family members who leave the workforce, either partially or completely, may be adversely affected. Women may be more adversely affected in this respect if the family decides that a man is earning a higher income, which it is preferable to retain.

Assuming, at least for the purpose of comparing costs, that a decent level of care were to be provided to those patients who were being placed in aged care, terminal, or whatever other description is applied, facilities it is difficult to see what extra costs would be imposed by caring for patients in a situation that permitted ongoing access by relatives involved in coma arousal programs.

The imposition of substantial costs on a community as a result of adoption of an untested therapy can be a valid reason for withholding an expensive new agent from widespread use before its efficacy has been established. It is, however, difficult to dress this argument up as a reason for requiring a randomised control trial before endorsing attempts by a patient's relatives to adopt an arousal program.

An economic rationalist might claim that participation in such a program was diverting resources away from productive use in the community. Productive use could occur if the family was free to make other contributions. If anyone were prepared seriously to present this argument, I believe that it might serve primarily to highlight the similarities between economic rationalism and coma.

A cynic might query whether opportunities for career advancement were coming into play as an outcome of the Westmead trial. The brief discussion above of the potential conflict between care of one's patient and inclusion of that patient in a trial may be relevant. It is worth noting that the majority of articles describing attempts to test the value of coma arousal programs retrieved in the Cochrane review *neither* met the criteria required at Westmead *nor* failed to be accepted for publication by reputable journals.

Passing from objections based on absence of randomisation and possible risks of a non-randomised trial without a simultaneous 'control' group, further objections were raised to the involvement of families in programs. The basis for these was that it would not be feasible to certify that all families were providing identical input. Resistance by some hospital doctors to family participation indicates a failure to recognise that Freeman's successes would have usually been unachievable without family insights, as shown in Roger's case in Chapter 2. Professional therapists complying with a generic protocol of stimulation would be unaware of such insights. It is similarly clear that their likely stimulatory impact, *as persons*, on the patients would be less than that of family members.

The notions of some hospital personnel about assessment of outcomes (namely, measurement of these after 10 weeks of a program) not only finally convinced the GIO to withdraw funding, but also indicated an ignorance of Freeman's earlier observations that led to the awarding of that grant. The outcomes of coma arousal programs clearly did not lend themselves to a school examination-type measurement indicating either 'pass' or 'fail'. Description in an earlier chapter of the 'soft signs' that were initially present intermittently and might only then be amenable to elicitation in familiar/familial surroundings should have alerted everyone to the need to tailor assessments individually and to repeat them. A school examination cannot be repeatedly undertaken in order to ensure that a true assessment of a candidate's ability is obtained: examination of a putatively comatose patient *must* be repeated to ensure its validity.

If the commitment of a group of comatose patients to a 'control'/non-treatment group is not acceptable, how could some assessment of the value of arousal programs have been achieved? One very practical suggestion, noted in Chapter 3, from an individual who had himself made a recovery from brain injury was that of a comparison with patients who had been 'warehoused' in terminal-care facilities following a brain injury. Such a comparison would, almost certainly, be politically unacceptable to any health minister.

An alternative, more politically palatable response could be to undertake a comparison of outcomes between two groups of patients, as closely matched as possible. One group would be people entered into active 'arousal' programs. Comparison could be with historical groups or with other contemporary groups receiving more conventional treatment. The discontinuation of the International Coma Data Bank removed one possibility for doing this.

A potentially viable alternative, suggested in 1995 by a medical practitioner who was a member of the NSW Parliament, was based on comparison of 'Freeman' patients with others entered into the State-wide system of Brain Injury Rehabilitation Program (BIRP) units, which operated in compliance with the accepted 'best practice' rehabilitation strategies.

The BIRP units dated from the late 1980s and were funded by the NSW Government through the Motor Accident Authority. Of 11 BIRP units established at that time, three were in the Sydney region and eight were located in country districts. In the mid 1990s, some academic rehabilitation specialists, in the course of developing an application for funding of a trial of coma arousal, considered the possibility of using outcome data from the BIRP system. At this time, it was discovered that this very well-funded system had not undertaken any study of the outcomes of its procedures. Furthermore, as will be mentioned in Chapter 7, there was trenchant opposition from BIRP practitioners to any involvement in such a comparative exercise. Their resistance to participation may have had a basis similar to their refusal to attend any meeting at which Freeman was present.

Another theoretically possible control group could have been derived from a coma register, had one existed. Freeman obtained agreement, in principle, to establish a register from a NSW health minister in the early 2000s but nothing eventuated.

The dispute between the GIO and the hospital, at the time when agreement was breaking down, over the duration of inclusion of any patient in the trial has been described above. It serves to highlight something that is a feature of any trial—namely, the nature of the assessment process that is to be utilised to generate the trial outcome data. This can vary considerably depending on what is being trialled.

Endpoints to a trial may be very clear—for example, death or survival. In the case of the Westmead trial, measurement of outcomes could, predictably, be seen not to be clear-cut. Neither the outcome for an individual patient nor the outcome of the aggregated patient group could be simply marked as pass or fail. The reasons for this difference relate to the gradual and often inconsistent course of emergence from coma, as discussed in Chapter 4.

Freeman's 'soft signs' might only be detectable intermittently at an early stage. They might only be observed separated in timing from the observer's attempt to elicit them by an interval sufficient to lead to a failure to recognise them as a response. Most importantly, they might, at least initially, only be demonstrable in the presence of family members. All of these requirements and limitations could easily be taken to invalidate observations made when adjusting for them.

It has been emphasised repeatedly that Freeman's success in assisting people was attributable to his recognition that communication was frequently dependent on the intermediation of family members. This applied equally whether the task was determining if a new patient was genuinely uncommunicative, deciding on the implementation of a stimulatory program or assessing whether a patient was emerging from coma after participating in a trial.

Conclusion

As with many of the events involving the management of people who remain unconscious for prolonged periods after brain injury, the history of this attempt to conduct a trial raises some general but crucial issues unrelated to brain injury.

It is axiomatic that, before its endorsement as an acceptable therapeutic response, any new treatment option should be trialled and shown to be at least as safe and effective as the forms of therapy already available. This entails the comparison of the new, 'experimental' therapy with the best existing 'control' therapy. That said, the specific form of trial to be adopted in any instance should be determined by the nature of that treatment. The epidemiological input to trial Freeman's approach to coma arousal recommended a double-blind randomised control format.

One feature of this format is that neither the practitioners responsible for the administration of the two types of therapy nor those undertaking the assessment of outcomes is aware of whether any participating subject is receiving the new therapy or the control one. The nature of the control will be determined by the types of therapies that already exist, but the control group is entitled to receive the best that is available. The randomisation referred to in the description of the trial refers to the allocation of entering subjects to either experimental or control groups. It is essential that entering subjects, or their representatives, consent to their random allocation to one of the groups.

It should have been evident from the outset of planning for the trial that this format was not compatible with the new form of therapy to be examined. There were both practical and ethical reasons for this. At a practical level, it would be impossible for either the supervising or the assessing medical practitioner to remain 'blinded' about which group of patients is receiving intensive stimulation from family members and which is receiving none. In view of the implicit wish of families requesting assistance from Freeman to receive this, it is not reasonable that any family, when adequately informed about the randomisation process, would be willing to risk being allocated to the control group. Most of the patients who were candidates for the trial had already experienced the 'control' process and found it to be inadequate. If genuinely informed consent—an ethical essential—had been required, there would have been no starters.

Passing from the issues of 'blinding' and informed consent that are applicable to any trial, there were some features peculiar to the proposed trial that would be incompatible with administration of therapy to the experimental group and measurement of outcomes in either group. An essential feature of Freeman's approach was the recruitment of people previously known to a patient to provide stimulation; however, if uniform stimulation was to be administered to all patients in the experimental group, the trial plan required that it be administered by paramedical personnel, an arrangement that would eliminate the availability of stimuli with personal relevance to the patient. In relation to measurement of outcomes, it was clear that early signs of awakening were commonly inconsistent ('soft signs'), and this would not readily slot into any reproducible scheme of recording.

All in all, the double-blind, randomised control trial format, whilst legitimately the backbone of any trial of a new drug, should have been seen to be quite inapplicable to a trial of coma arousal. One size, clearly, does not fit all. This incompatibility has been demonstrated by the absence of any trial that has fully met the criteria of the Cochrane study for this trial format.

Additional impediments, if any were needed, to the trial being accomplished were the scepticism of some of the personnel involved, the collision between determination of when a patient exited the trial to enter the hospital's rehabilitation program and the lure of the relatively large budget of the trial.

Leaving aside consideration of the format of the trial, some of its features would have been difficult to accommodate within the general aims of trials. Any trial is required to determine that the new therapy under test is both at least as safe as established alternatives and at least as effective as the alternatives (but, preferably, better). In practice, the first of these requirements would usually imply that the 'experimental' group could be at a disadvantage, but, in the proposed trial, it was much more likely that the control group who were receiving the established therapy would be disadvantaged by deprivation of access to the new therapy. The reason for this was that the established form of therapy was acknowledged by hospital personnel to be effectively 'no treatment'.

Apart from the impediments considered above, the events during the lead-up to implementation of the trial raised some disturbing questions about potential conflicts of interest between the dual role of participating doctors as clinicians and as researchers. On some occasions, it appeared that, when dealing with experimental subjects, the research aspirations of the clinicians with this dual responsibility could be trumping their responsibilities to the same individuals as patients.

7. Concerted opposition in Australia

The events described in the two preceding chapters—namely, the evolution of Freeman's ideas and practice on domiciliary rehabilitation and the machinations evoked by the availability of a large grant of research funding—occurred against a background of considerable hostility towards those ideas and practices. The extent to which this general hostility fuelled the antagonism expressed in individual situations and happenings is not readily discernible after a quarter-century. Similarly, questions about the relative contributions of various influences to the development and entrenchment of the opposition are not easily resolved. This chapter recounts a sample of the hostile responses from some Australian medical personnel. The next chapter balances this against international support for Freeman's ideas, frequently forthcoming as a reaction to the attacks described below.

At the outset, it appears fairly clear that opposition originated among Freeman's medical colleagues. Expressions of opposition in the context of the health system at large can be traced back, with some confidence, to a relatively small number of members of the medical profession. Opposition to Freeman was not generalised within the profession, but critics were considerably more vocal than supporters. The Australian Medical Association, of which Freeman was a member, was supportive of him. There were clinical leaders within the profession who, while not necessarily endorsing chapter and verse of Freeman's thinking, considered that his clinical observations were potentially of major significance and merited an open-minded assessment.

One issue that was raised in criticisms of Freeman related to the paucity of laboratory data, derived from experimental systems, pointing to some superiority of his active early approach to patient rehabilitation. This argument failed, and continues to fail, to take account of two other issues. The first of these was the almost total lack of hard laboratory data supporting the prevailing approach of non-intervention. The second was the obstinacy implicit in discounting clinical observations that Freeman's approach appeared to help some patients and harmed none.

Following his visit to the United States in 1983, Freeman sought advice from the Director of the John Curtin School of Medical Research at The Australian National University:

> Bob Porter had a reputation as an international neuroscientist. I told him about the research on brain injury. I spoke about the nerve cells sprouting like buds on the branch of a tree. He listened for half an hour and suggested that I should not become involved in studying the brain at the cellular level, but should demonstrate what could be done with the patients.

The advice was taken.

As already suggested in discussing the aborted trial at the Westmead Hospital, a factor specific to that episode is likely to have contributed to moves to exclude Freeman from the process. In short, it would require a combination of exceptional naivety and charity not to indict a strong motivation to appropriate the funding offered by the GIO as an important factor in that attempted exclusion.

As to the more general factors fuelling opposition, apprehension about considering therapeutic proposals that were very much at odds with accepted practice was certainly important. A distinction should, however, be drawn between exercising caution about accepting, let alone adopting, practices contrary to established precepts and refusing at least to consider new ideas and give their proponents an uninterrupted hearing. The former is prudent, the latter prejudiced.

Another contributing factor, albeit an unproven one, to opposition to Freeman and his ideas may have been the realisation that any degree of acceptance of them must implicitly be a criticism of the then prevailing management of people with substantial brain injuries. 'Management' is used here in its broadest medical sense. Thus, Freeman persistently challenged *diagnoses* made by his colleagues. He persistently issued *prognoses* that, although heavily guarded, retained possibilities of hopeful outcomes. As a result of his diagnosis and prognosis, he persistently recommended rehabilitation *treatment* that was heavily dependent on contributions from families and communities rather than on professionals.

For all of these reasons, he was condemned by specific groups of colleagues—namely, those whose responsibilities entailed the acute care of individuals with brain injury and those responsible for their rehabilitation. The first group often regarded his intervention at the behest of families as a direct attack on their diagnostic competence. A recovery, even with substantial persisting disability, could be read as such an assertion. The second group, with responsibility for rehabilitation of people with brain injuries, found Freeman's willingness to assist patients who had been categorised as unsuitable for rehabilitation offensive.

Exclusion

Opposition to Freeman on the part of particular colleagues was expressed in many ways. Perhaps the most childish was to restrict his access to patients whom their families had asked him to visit. In some instances, his visit to a hospital was met with studied officiousness. An example of this in a NSW hospital occurred when Freeman, at the request of a patient's wife, and with prior agreement from the neurosurgeon and the hospital, arrived at the hospital: He records:

I was surprised to be asked to go to the office of the Director of Medical Services. I waited outside for an excessively long time before being invited into the room of the director, who asked me to sit down. She questioned me about what I wanted to do at the hospital and then asked me, 'Can you show me your medical registration?' I did so. She asked, 'Can you show me documents that you are in the medical defence?' I did so. She asked, 'Would you show me your driver's licence?' I thought this was a peculiar request but complied. Next she asked to see two credit cards. I produced them. She then asked, 'Would you show me your passport?' I thought this was totally out of order, but replied, 'I do not usually carry my passport with me. Why do you ask?' The director said, 'I will give you permission on this occasion to see the patient, but we do not like having you in this hospital.'

Freeman gave an account of this episode to a colleague, a former federal president of the Australian Medical Association, whose response was 'silly bloody idiot'. Whilst Freeman regarded the director as a particularly rude person, his commitment was to visit the patient, not to argue with the director.

At other times, he was left in no doubt that his future presence was not welcomed. An example of this tactic was the response to Freeman's visit to the patient Donald recounted in Chapter 2. Freeman described the circumstances after he had examined Donald:

The Neurosurgical Registrar, when I had completed my examination, walked to the ward door with me and said, 'I have been told to tell you—we don't want you to come back.' I asked why, but he ignored me.

Sometimes, Freeman was refused any access to a patient despite parental requests. In the case of Louise, a young woman who had suffered a severe brain injury and was likely to be sent to a nursing home, he recalled:

As the hospital authorities were reluctant to allow me entry into the hospital ward, Sister Jeanette Budak arranged for Louise's parents to bring her in a wheelchair into the hospital car park for assessment. A car park is not the best or most private place to assess a patient but at least Louise had remained on hospital premises. Immediately I saw this young lady, I knew that she had awareness.

Following the attack on him in the NSW Parliament, described later in this chapter, exclusion of Freeman from hospitals was directed from levels higher than that of hospital administrators. On one occasion, the parents of a boy with a severe brain injury who had requested the hospital management to permit Freeman to examine their son received a reply from the NSW Department of Health as follows:

Unfortunately as Dr Freeman is not accredited to attend patients at ... Hospital he would not be able to see your son on this basis. As Dr Freeman has a different philosophy for those with traumatic brain injury there have been several occasions where different methods of treatment have caused conflict. I understand your concerns and need to explore every avenue but at this stage it is not feasible to agree to your request.

Another manifestation of opposition was the exclusion of Freeman from presentations and projects concerned with management of brain injury. These exclusions contrast with the invitations which, paradoxically, Freeman was concurrently receiving to participate in international conferences as the sole Australian invitee.

In July 1987, the NSW Government introduced a new transport accident compensation scheme, Transcover. The new scheme was intended to replace the existing arrangement under which the injured person received a single lump-sum compensation payment with ongoing financial support that could fund continuing rehabilitation. To mark this change, a seminar was arranged and, as severe brain injury was the commonest condition requiring prolonged rehabilitation, the seminar was devoted to this subject. Freeman was invited to attend and, given his commitment to continuing rehabilitation, he assumed that he would be programmed as a speaker. He was, however, disabused some weeks before the seminar when visited by the GIO official responsible for organising it. In Freeman's words:

> When we sat down over a cup of coffee he said, 'I am sorry, Ted, but you will not be invited to speak.' He appeared to be embarrassed. 'Why not?' I asked. 'Because other speakers will not stand on the same platform if you participate.' I was astonished—in my opinion, this was not an objective scientific attitude in response to a major community health problem—but obviously John felt that he was in an extremely difficult position. He said he could not risk my inclusion because it had been a major effort to push the NSW Government to agree to Transcover.

The speakers at the seminar were to be two persons from a consultancy speaking on the Transcover scheme, two participants from the abandoned Westmead study speaking on research on brain injury rehabilitation and two rehabilitation specialists both of whom had been critics of Freeman's approach.

Abandoned research proposals

In the following year, a leading neurosurgeon in Victoria advised Freeman that he was attempting to initiate a study of coma arousal in that State. He advised

Freeman that he had shown his book on coma to some neurosurgeons and 'they took exception to the fact that I was encouraging families to "impose" their own ideas on the treatment of their relative'. Freeman's correspondent continued that, according to the neurosurgeons, 'the whole thing was hopelessly unscientific'. He concluded: 'I finally end up with a list of who will cooperate and who won't. One minute all is sweetness and light, and the next there are innumerable difficulties.'[1] Predictably, the study was abandoned.

History was to repeat itself 10 years later. As mentioned in the preceding chapter, a medical practitioner who was a member of the NSW Parliament proposed to the then health minister that it would be appropriate to undertake a review of Ted Freeman's work on rehabilitation following brain injury. Coincidentally, research psychologist Dr Ross Harris, an expert in pain management, together with a rehabilitation specialist holding a university appointment who had consistently perceived value in that work, had been preparing, at the request of the National Brain Injury Foundation, a protocol for a research project, tentatively titled the Brain Injury Outcome Study (BIOS).

In order to initiate the BIOS, some means of accessing a historical control group of patients with brain injury who had been treated by 'conventional' procedures would provide a baseline. The best source of such data seemed to be the outcomes achieved to that time by the NSW Brain Injury Rehabilitation Program (BIRP). Information from the BIRP units could then provide a baseline for comparison with data relating to community rehabilitation.

As noted in the previous discussion of clinical trials, when a request was made, through a government body, the Motor Accident Authority, for access to the outcome statistics from the BIRP, it emerged that, notwithstanding very adequate funding over a number of years, no statistics had been collected. Apparently, the BIRP units had not been sufficiently concerned with assessing the efficacy of their unchallenged practices to undertake simple statistical collection or evaluation. For example, no information was available as to which forms of therapy had been most successful when provided to different groups of patients with brain injuries. The irony of this was not lost on Ted Freeman:

> Over the years of my involvement in the field of brain injury some of the directors of BIRP units, most of whom I had never met, had been highly critical of my approach to the treatment of brain injury, accusing me of having no scientific basis for my work. None had ever corresponded with me about my medical papers, which had been published in refereed international journals, and none had acknowledged or rejected the theories advanced in my book on coma.

---

1   Keith Henderson, Letter to Freeman, November 1989.

Antagonism to Freeman and his procedures, it turned out, was not a thing of the past, even in 1997. Notwithstanding the lack of records from the preceding decade, the current practice within the BIRP units could have provided control data for a contemporary assessment of Freeman's practices. The research psychologist who was seeking to undertake a comparative assessment of Freeman's ideas and the generally prevailing practices in New South Wales realised that this could only be possible if the BIRP units were participating. Yet antagonism to Freeman remained alive and well. In attempting to secure participation by some BIRP units, the specialist arranged meetings with the directors. It soon became abundantly clear to him that, if Freeman was invited to participate in any of these meetings, the directors would boycott them. The specialist was effectively in a lose–lose situation.

An ideal approach to establishing a comparative study of the efficacy of 'established' and 'Freeman' procedures was envisaged as entering a group of patients, who had already been classified as 'not suitable for rehabilitation' by a BIRP unit, into a community-based rehabilitation program. The most cursory rereading of the patient stories in Chapters 2 and 3 indicates that many of Freeman's patients during the preceding two decades had met this criterion and had indeed been so diagnosed. They had been, in all but formal naming, the 'rejects' of the system. In contrast with this history, when the rehabilitation specialist met with BIRP unit directors, his meeting notes recorded:

[T]here is a difficulty in that no-one will commit to paper that in their opinion a particular patient is 'not suitable for rehabilitation'.

Apart from the resistance of the BIRP unit directors to participation in any study of Freeman's outcomes, the BIOS was doomed by the resource allocation approved by the NSW Government. The arrangement would be that the BIRP units would continue to receive considerable funding, as in the past, to undertake their programs and the university-based BIOS would receive the resources required to undertake the study. In contrast, the patients entered into community-based rehabilitation would be dependent on *minimal guidance and education*.

Freeman interpreted 'minimal guidance and education' as a deliberate attempt to ensure the failure of that part of the research that was supposed to be evaluating the community-based program. Needless to say, the BIOS did not commence.

At this juncture, it should be repeated that opposition to anything connected with Ted Freeman was certainly not universal among the medical community, or even among the specialist neurological and neurosurgical subpopulations within that community. Whilst a number of senior practitioners were prepared to confide to Freeman that they perceived merit, at least partial, in his ideas and their practical application, a much smaller group was prepared to state this publicly. An even smaller group was prepared to express support for the testing of his practices after initially opposing them. This required an open mind—not necessarily a given within the profession.

Formal opposition

Apart from individual initiatives to exclude Freeman from the medical community as in the examples above, some collective attacks were mounted. In May 1986, the Australian Association of Neurologists (AAN) wrote to the federal health minister to express its concerns in the following terms:[2]

> You may be aware that 'coma arousal' is a name given to a very active rehabilitation of head injured patients. A unit has been active in Sydney for some time and those involved with the unit claim that 'coma arousal' achieves more than the simple passage of time and traditional physical therapies.

The association asserted that the treatment was costly and, perhaps providing an indication of the motivation underlying the letter (the trial at the Westmead Hospital had lost its GIO funding at the end of the preceding year), continued: 'there appears to have been a reluctance on the part of those proposing this therapy for it to be submitted to appropriately controlled scientific trials.'

In June 1987, the National Health and Medical Research Council (NHMRC), the premier body charged with overseeing Australian medical research, weighed into the attack. As had been the case with the AAN letter to the minister, no prior attempt was made to consult with the Australian Brain Foundation, a well-credentialled body that had been backing Freeman's approach to rehabilitation, or with Freeman himself. At the 103rd session of the Council:

> Council noted that coma arousal therapy, an as yet unproven therapeutic modality used on severely brain injured persons, continues to be actively promoted. In addition, it was noted that there are considerable psychosocial implications for relatives and close friends of patients for whom this treatment may be suggested.

> While the mobilisation of hope is part of such programs they may lead to unrealistic expectations with problems for family functioning, guilt and grief. Thus a thorough evaluation of positive and negative outcomes in a controlled trial is essential.

---

2   Correspondence, Australian Association of Neurologists to the Minister for Health, 20 May 1986.

Council expressed the view that new forms of treatment should not be promoted unless supported by the results of scientifically valid clinical trials.

In the case of coma arousal therapy such a trial should be practically and ethically possible. Council accepted that the rehabilitation of head injured patients is a problem of major concern in our society and expressed the opinion that the development of scientific trials of new treatment modalities in this area is to be strongly encouraged and supported.[3]

Two points claimed by the NHMRC disclose some ignorance on its part concerning the subject on which it was pontificating. In the first instance, the 'considerable psychological implications' and 'unrealistic explanations' that it cited had already been studied by a Macquarie University research team with results that were entirely favourable to the practice of Freeman's group and quite dismissive of the NHMRC's envisaged concerns. Although that study was funded by the GIO, rather than by the NHMRC itself, it would be entirely reasonable to expect that the council staffer preparing the advice, which was patently based on unpublished opinion, might also have been aware of unpublished research at a major Australian university that contradicted the argument it presented.

A second issue, on which one might have hoped that the council should have been more knowledgeable, relates to the assertion that a trial should be 'practically and ethically possible'. As the Cochrane review of the practicality of similar trials was to discover two decades later, it had not proved possible to complete a statistically acceptable study complying with the generic guidelines for randomised control trials. One of the responsibilities of the NHMRC is that of maintaining ethical overview of all medical research projects in the nation, irrespective of their funding source. Given this, it is rather disappointing that those advising the Council had not been able to discern the massive ethical quandaries inherent in trials of the type of the failed Westmead one. Freeman wrote to the NHMRC Chair with a detailed rebuttal of the claims in the recommendations in September 1987 but failed to receive a reply. Even in 1987, the Australian community was entitled to expect better from its peak medical research body.

A postscript to these events affords an interesting perspective on the manner in which collective mind-sets survive even as history overtakes them. A 1995 request from the NSW branch of the Australian Medical Association to the NHMRC for a meeting to examine Freeman's practices and outcomes brought

---

3   National Health and Medical Research Council, 103rd Session, June 1987.

the response from the Chairman of the NHMRC that '[t]he position on coma arousal therapy as discussed in June 1987 is still current and there is no plan to review it at present'.

Had the Chairman's mind been sufficiently open to seek some wider advice, he would have found that Freeman was, at the time of the request for an examination of his activities, in London participating in PVS 95, a small, invited group of international specialists examining methods of facilitating rehabilitation after brain injury. Some detail about this meeting will be included in the next chapter, which discusses some international assessments of Freeman's achievements.

Pilloried in Parliament

All of the preceding attacks on Freeman shrank in perspective when he became the victim of a defamatory attack under parliamentary privilege. When placed in historical context, this can be seen as one of the most despicable abuses of privilege in an institution that is no stranger to that practice.

In 1988, Ted Freeman was asked by Gail and Rollyn Graham to meet with their son Jim, who remained severely disabled as a result of a brain injury five years previously. Jim's parents had worked unremittingly over that period attempting to obtain the best possible outcome for him. This had included a period in a US clinic, admissions to a succession of Australian hospitals and an ongoing correspondence with those administering health care, not to mention politicians. Gail has written a book giving an account of the problems that she and Rollyn encountered and this has attracted widespread attention.

After Ted Freeman had been approached to assist Jim, Gail circulated to every member of the NSW Parliament a letter outlining the obstacles that the Graham family had encountered. Recipients included the health minister and his opposition shadow. Whilst many members replied to her letter, this pair failed to do so. Prophetically, Gail wrote about the health minister, Peter Collins, 'he can't ignore us forever'. This proved to be correct. On 9 February 1989, the minister wrote to all Legislative Assembly members acknowledging receipt of the Grahams' representations on the subject, stating that the Health Department had 'reacted appropriately by investigating details of this patient and communicating with his mother. Further assessment of his condition and the need for future treatment has been offered.'

Gail Graham has written of this ministerial action:

> We were speechless. Except for one odd phone call, nobody from Mr Collins' department had communicated with either of us. Certainly no

further assessment of Jim's needs had been offered. Nothing whatsoever had been offered. Worst of all Jim's situation had been misrepresented to the only people who were in a position to help us.[4]

Ted Freeman's unpublished account of what eventuated, as communicated by Gail Graham, follows:

> Gail and Rollyn were extremely frustrated in their attempts to make contact with Collins so they made huge posters that said 'Why won't you talk to us Mr Collins', and stationed themselves on the footpath outside the NSW Parliament House. Soon a member of staff approached them on the footpath and told them that, if they removed the posters, they could have a meeting with Collins that afternoon. Gail recorded the interview. In it Collins turned his back on her and spoke only to Rollyn. Collins prevented Rollyn from completing his sentences. Collins blamed the Federal Government for Jim's predicament. The meeting finished with Collins saying he would be speaking about the matter in Parliament two weeks later, on 1 March 1989.

Concurrently with the initiatives of Gail and Rollyn Graham, the Brain Injury Division of the Australian Brain Foundation had been preparing a submission to the NSW Health Department requesting funding for a study of coma arousal. Essentially, this proposed that 20 patients who had been diagnosed as 'vegetative' or 'unfit for rehabilitation' in hospitals would be transferred to the Brain Injury Therapy Centre at Eastwood. These patients would be assessed at regular intervals by independent medical examiners. After the proposal was submitted to the Health Department, the Australian Brain Foundation learned that a favourable response was possible and that (coincidentally) the minister would be making a statement on the subject to Parliament on 1 March 1989.

At 2.30 pm on the appointed day, the minister rose from his seat to address the Legislative Assembly. *Hansard* records the following:

> *Mr Collins:* I am concerned that the Grahams have circulated misleading correspondence to many members of Parliament—

> (interruption)

> *Speaker:* Order!

> *Mr Collins:* —suggesting that neither Jim's doctors at Mt Wilga, the Department of Health, nor my staff have offered any assistance. This is incorrect.

> (interruption)

---

4   Gail Graham (1995) *Staying Alive*. Angus & Robertson, Sydney.

Speaker: Order! Having had three general calls to order, I call the honourable member for Waverley and ask the Serjeant-at-Arms to remove him. (The honourable member for Waverley, Mr Ernie Page, left the chamber accompanied by the Serjeant-at-Arms.)

Following this diversion, the minister proceeded to read from a document.

Mr Collins: Dr Freeman has over a number of years sought government endorsement for his therapeutic approach—commonly called coma arousal therapy. The Government Insurance Office in a report by Cuff Consultants to the previous Government issued the following advice about Dr Freeman:

This report which I shall later seek to table is dated the 6th March 1987. It continues:

The therapy centre is not legitimate research work.

The therapy centre activity does not constitute rehabilitation of brain injured people and their families.

The therapy centre activity has not improved disability outcomes despite the relatively high cost.

There are questions of medical and professional ethics in regard to the division's activities.

Dr Freeman is not conducting his work within any scientific framework. He does not even try to respond to requests for justification of his concepts or beliefs: he seems totally unconcerned about the rightness or wrongness of his ideas.

The Brain Injury Therapy Centre is not staffed for the rehabilitation of brain injury. Dr Freeman does not assess the patients in the objective manner required by the rehabilitation process to measure both the recovery and the effectiveness of the rehabilitation effort. The medical practices preferred by the Brain Injury Therapy Centre are unacceptable to rehabilitation professionals particularly as they are performed on helpless people unprotected by any legislation.

Continuing to read from the Cuff Report, the minister quoted from the NHMRC recommendation described above and followed with:

In 1984–5 the doctor withdrew from a joint GIO–Westmead Hospital study aimed at assessing coma arousal.

The minister concluded his statement making reference to the Grahams:

The Grahams, like other parents in this heart wrenching position, should take some consolation in that they have done everything possible for their child—so too will health workers in our public health care system who continue caring for young Jim Graham.

Aftermath of the parliamentary attack

Reactions to the Collins statement were profound. Ted Freeman decided to retire, hoping that criticism of him would then have less unfavourable impact on the BITC. He has recalled the time immediately after the minister's statement:

> *On the afternoon of 1 March 1989, after the Minister for Health, the Hon. Peter Collins, had made his speech in the NSW Legislative Assembly, I left Parliament House and walked down Macquarie Street in a state of shock and bewilderment. This was not the outcome I had expected. I wondered why the proposal to research 20 patients labelled as 'vegetative' or 'unsuitable for rehabilitation' had been rejected. Weighing heavily on my mind was the fact that to be publicly criticised in Parliament by the Minister for Health could ruin the professional reputation of any doctor, and I was aware that now it might be impossible for me to continue my work in the field of brain injury.*

The Grahams were very distressed. Gail has written an account in her book:

> We were both devastated. In particular Rollyn felt that he had been personally humiliated, because on top of everything else, Peter Collins had publicly rebuked him. He said that now people would think it was his fault that Jim was being denied the treatment he needed. Jim probably thought so too, Rollyn said. This was ridiculous but nothing that I [Gail] or anybody else could say seemed to comfort him. He became convinced that his colleagues and students were talking about him behind his back, laughing at him, holding him in contempt.[5]

Two weeks later, Rollyn committed suicide.

As mentioned above, consternation raged among the families of people under treatment at the Brain Injury Therapy Centre. The Brain Injury Division of the Australian Brain Foundation was disbanded. The BITC administration was reshaped in an attempt to overcome the impact of the statement. With Freeman no longer having any position in the BITC, it was replaced with a more commercially oriented venture, Brain Injury Services Proprietary Limited, led

---

5   Ibid.

by an entrepreneurial executive. Within a year of its formation, this company was liquidated in circumstances characterised by the accountants as entailing 'gross mismanagement, profligate and irrational expenditure and also, it appears, nepotism'. The liquidator concluded that none of the medical staff associated with the BITC had been aware of any financial impropriety or mismanagement.

The Sydney tabloid press on the following day ran headlines drawn from the liquidator's findings, effectively compounding the damage previously done to community perceptions of coma arousal.

The Cuff Report examined

As the devastation of lives following Collins' statement of March 1989 derived from conclusions of the Cuff Report included in that statement, it is appropriate to formulate some assessment of the quality of that report. As the Report became a public document after the statement, this is not difficult. Answers to the questions of why the report was only released two years after its completion, of its location during that interval and of who was pulling the strings to bring it to the minister's attention before any of the people attacked in it were given an opportunity to comment are less easily answered.

The story of the commissioning of the Report is as follows. In 1986, the GIO was preparing for legislative changes to enable the conversion of the existing practice of single compensation payouts into structured settlements whereby the insurance company provided an annuity on a set pay scale for life, depending on the extent of the patient's disability. As a first step, the necessity to determine the extent and cost to the community of severe brain injury was acknowledged. A GIO official wrote a detailed letter in September 1986 outlining the problems to Chris Cuff, of Cuff Management Consultants, with a request: 'What I am now seeking is your assistance in pulling together all these issues and determining strategies for future GIO involvement and for the establishment of a new study on the treatment of the brain injured.'

A report was presented to the GIO Third Party Division on 6 March 1987.[6]

When refereeing an article's suitability for acceptance in a medical publication, one would be provided with some indication of relevant qualifications or professional position held by the author. As the only attribution of authorship disclosed in the Report is 'Cuff Consultants', it is reasonable, given the nature of its content, to assume some expertise on the part of the author(s) and then

---

6   Cuff Consultants (1987) *Report on the Brain Injury Division. Presentation to GIO Third Party Division*, 6 March 1987.

to proceed to review it as one would deal with an article on rehabilitation after brain injury emanating from an appropriately qualified source. The authority which was accorded the Report conferred by its parliamentary release permits of no other conclusion.

The Report contains a number of sections, each of which is headlined with the conclusion derived from it, followed by the information on which that conclusion has been based. In order to provide a basis for its evaluation, each conclusion will be cited. Following this, an abbreviated account of the supporting information contained in the report is provided. A critique of each conclusion and its supporting information, including comments referring to it from several independent healthcare practitioners, follows.

Freeman's theories disparaged

The first two conclusions concern the nature of the theories underlying Freeman's practices, and do not consider the clinical outcomes of those practices.

• Ted Freeman's treatment of severely disabled people seems to be based on a 'triad' of concepts/beliefs about the ability of the brain to regain function; none of these beliefs has the validation of any scientific evidence.

• Specialists in the rehabilitation of brain-injured people have asked Ted Freeman to explain the basis and nature of his ideas.

The three concepts identified in the supporting information attached to the first conclusion relate to the ability of the brain to repair itself or to compensate for loss following injury. They are 'the plasticity of the brain', 'the spare capacity of the brain' and 'canalisation—the inherent fixed pathway of recovery'. In the report's discussion of these, the first two are dismissed as having 'no scientific validation', whilst the third is dismissed as 'pure conjecture'.

No attribution of a credible scientific source for the dismissal of these three theories is provided in the Report. No evidence has been presented in the Report to support these conclusions. The Report will be examined only in the light of what was generally accepted in 1987 and so will not, for example, assess it in the light of the more recent universal acceptance of the reality of neuroplasticity. A commentary informed by some knowledge of the state of experimental neuroscience in 1987 might have concluded that little was known, on the basis of experimentation, *either for or against* the three concepts. They remained to be tested in experimental models; however, given the available clinical observations pointing to them at the time of the report, each constituted a reasonable hypothesis.

The second conclusion is supported by a claim that Freeman had failed to respond to questions about his proposals for rehabilitating patients who remain unconscious following brain injuries. Whilst the Report's conclusion, presented above, refers to 'specialists', the supporting information relates only to input from a single practitioner. This takes the form of a copy of a letter sent to Freeman by the clinical superintendent of an Adelaide clinic undertaking rehabilitation of patients after brain injury. The copied letter has been highlighted in 22 places at each of which its author is said to have directed questions to Freeman. All questions are said to refer to points made by Freeman in his papers, either published or in draft form (it would be unusual for an author to pass the latter to hostile colleagues before publication). As no attempt is made in the supporting information to disguise the existence of an antagonistic relationship between Freeman and the writer of the letter, one might question its objectivity.

Reference to Freeman's publication list reveals that his writings were invariably published in peer-reviewed journals, usually internationally based. Consequently, it is probable that many, if not all, of the points that have been queried by the Adelaide doctor had been accepted and approved as reasonable statements by unbiased overseas professionals qualified in the field of brain injury. If referees had challenged any, Freeman would have been required either to amend them or to justify their inclusion to the satisfaction of the journal editor before acceptance of a manuscript for publication. The scrutiny to which Freeman's presentation of his ideas had been subjected before their acceptance in the scientific literature contrasts with the lack of anything resembling scientific process in the discussion of possible theories in the report.

It may be appropriate to balance the comments of the Adelaide-based practitioner on Freeman's work with the inclusion of those of two extremely well-qualified, senior, Adelaide academic clinicians.

Professor Donald Simpson, Professor of Neurosurgery at the University of Adelaide, wrote in March 1989 after the parliamentary attack on Freeman: 'One of the merits of Freeman's work is that it has stimulated an overall improvement in rehabilitation services and he has played a respectable role in the development of rehabilitation in Australia.'[7]

Dr Roger Rees, Director of the Institutes for Learning Difficulties in Adelaide (subsequently Professor of Disability Studies and Research at Flinders University, Adelaide), wrote, also in March 1989:

> The Brain Therapy Centre at Eastwood has undertaken pioneering intervention with some of the most severely brain injured persons in Australia. The team work approach allied to the persistence is unique

---

7   Donald Simpson, Letter to Freeman, March 1989.

and can best occur when the therapy unit also provides a social network which acts as a life-raft for the brain injured and their families. The Brain Injury Therapy Centre at Eastwood provides a state of the art program which meets an important need for long term individual therapy and family support for persons with severe disability.[8]

Freeman's clinical competence attacked

Three of the conclusions in the Report amount to criticisms of Freeman as a clinician. These are considered individually, together with their supporting arguments and an evaluation of each. The first was:

- Rehabilitation specialists take responsibility for prognosis in regard to patients' disabilities and consequent needs: Ted Freeman does not take this responsibility.

In support of this contention, the Cuff Report compares two responses to legal requests on prognosis. Both have been selected from GIO files. One of these is headed as 'typical' while the other response is attributed to Ted Freeman. Whilst this is not explicitly stated, the second response is, presumably, intended to be 'typical' of Freeman. It relates to a request from the GIO to which the report's authors can find no answer in the file.

Any decent assessment of Freeman's response to requests from solicitors should consider factors such as the comparability of the relationship to the specific patient of Freeman and the 'typical' rehabilitation practitioner. For example, had Freeman examined that patient once or twice whilst the 'typical' practitioner had full clinical responsibility for an inpatient on a daily basis? A reasonable comparison would necessarily be based on a comprehensive examination of the records of many patients. The second conclusion of the Report was:

- Ted Freeman does not assess the progress of patients in the objective manner required by the rehabilitation process to measure both recovery and the effectiveness of the rehabilitation process.

This conclusion was supported by a comparison between Freeman's approach to assessment and that undertaken at the Prince Henry Hospital Rehabilitation Unit. As with the preceding comparison, a single 'Freeman' patient is used as an information source. The Prince Henry Hospital assessment method required the allocation of a numerical score to indicate a patient's status as measured for a number of functions. For example, the first two functions to be estimated were 'mental capacity' and 'psychological activities' and the rehabilitation specialist

---

8   Roger Rees, Letter to Freeman, March 1989.

was required to allocate a score within a range of 1–12 and 1–6 respectively. For comparison, Freeman's assessment of a specific patient included descriptions, without any attempt at attaching a numerical scale, to categories such as 'emotion' and 'independence of drive'.

Admittedly, the allocation of numbers to a patient's estimated competence will permit aggregation of results achieved in a group of patients and one can derive means, standard errors, and so on. With great respect to social scientists, however, the question that a more competent report author might have asked is that of whether converting assessment of an entity such as 'emotion' to a numerical value actually achieves much other than camouflaging something that is no more than a subjective estimate. Freeman's description of his patients, I submit, conveys much more information to someone wishing to know about their status. The third conclusion of the Report was:

- Ted Freeman does not have the concern of people with long experience in the rehabilitation of brain-injured people in regard to the needs of families.

This criticism of Freeman's clinical practice is sourced to three concerned, anonymous commentators who deplore his lack of awareness of the needs of patients' families.

A quick reread of Chapter 3 containing families' firsthand accounts of their experiences with Freeman will shed some light on this one. Unfortunately, these letters were not written until the mid 1990s, so could not be seen by the three anonyms. But wait. The Macquarie University study that was concerned precisely with the impact of their association with Freeman on patients' families had been completed by December 1986 (see Chapter 6). This study was funded by the GIO, so its conclusions—very different from those asserted in the conclusion above—would have been accessible to the Report's authors. Given the evident access to GIO files provided to Cuff Consultants, it would be surprising if the authors of the Report were unaware of the conclusions of the Macquarie study. These emphatically refuted the opinions of the three individuals, which provided the basis for this third Report conclusion criticising Freeman's clinical performance.

The Brain Injury Treatment Centre's practices attacked

Whereas the three critical conclusions discussed above related to Freeman as a person, three other adverse conclusions advanced by Cuff Consultants focused on the structure and operations of the BITC. The first was:

- The rehabilitation of people with brain injury involves skills from many disciplines; the rehabilitation process assists both the person and responsible relatives.

The supporting information accompanying this conclusion outlines the variety of skills and resources available to a young woman who had sustained a brain injury, after she had been admitted to the Coorabel Rehabilitation Hospital (this information was presented preparatory to comparison with those skills and resources provided at the BITC).

The striking difference between this outline and the role of the BITC is that the young woman had been admitted to Coorabel as soon as she was no longer in need of ventilator support, some 20 days after sustaining the brain injury. As the most cursory familiarity with the BITC should have revealed, patients admitted to it were not 'fresh' but had previously spent long periods either with little progress, in 'orthodox' rehabilitation facilities, or stored in some type of prolonged-care facility. To express this more crudely, Freeman's patients were invariably 'rejects' not suitable for any(more) orthodox rehabilitation. They had not been regarded as 'suitable for rehabilitation'. Consequently, they had usually been denied access to 'conventional' programs incorporating the multidisciplinary skills on offer at Coorabel.

In relation to this point, a senior lecturer in neurology at the University of Sydney, Dr Michael Halmagyi, who had visited the centre, wrote of the Report that the critics were not in possession of the facts:

> [V]irtually none of the critics have been to the Centre or spoken with any of its patients. If it had not been for Ted Freeman's work, more brain injured people would be warehoused and the brain injury problem would have been largely ignored by the government.[9]

Dr Halmagyi provided an excellent example of a practitioner who was prepared to keep an open mind when confronted with new information that was not readily explained. He had originally been critical of Freeman's approach to rehabilitation, in the course of a radio interview, but had accepted an invitation to visit the centre. Freeman recalled, in relation to the visit, that

> *as we walked around looking at the family and staff and volunteers working with these most profoundly brain injured patients, I could see that he was moved by their plight and the care and concern with which they were being treated. He came back to my room and said, 'Something must be done to help these people.' He offered his support.*

---

9   Michael Halmagyi, Letter cited in press release from Professional Public Relations, 2 March 1989.

A second adverse report conclusion is directed to the purported inadequacies of the BITC:

- The Brain Injury Therapy Centre is not staffed for the rehabilitation of brain injury.

This report conclusion is supported by a comparison of staff profiles at Coorabel and at another head injury rehabilitation institution with those of the BITC. Details of bed capacity for which staff had responsibility at the three institutions were not provided. No indication was given as to the comparability of the patient profile. To attempt any comparison between institutions, information such as time elapsed since injury and preceding management of residents is essential. Whereas both Coorabel and the SA facility had many more specialised paramedical staff, the BITC lists 10 registered nurses and three assistant nurses. Coorabel lists 'nurses' without any numbers. The other facility under comparison does not list any.

Without knowing the needs of typical patients in the facilities, and the aggregate workload that they would generate, it is difficult to derive much from this comparison. As remarked in the preceding critique, Freeman's patients consisted primarily of people who had not made it into the rehabilitation programs to which the cited staffing profiles related. During the interval between discharge from acute care until entry to the BITC, they are unlikely to have been in receipt of the attention provided by 'mainstream' rehabilitation. The third adverse conclusion claimed:

- The medical practices preferred by the Brain Injury Therapy Centre are unacceptable to rehabilitation professionals, particularly as they are performed on helpless people unprotected by any legislation.

This section presents brief descriptions of alleged incorrect/inappropriate procedures undertaken under Ted Freeman's auspices, presumably in the BITC. No attribution of the source(s) of these descriptions was provided.

This conclusion hints at the occurrence of illegal practices of which residents of the BITC were the victims. If improper practices are alleged to have occurred at the BITC, they should have been raised with the authorities responsible for oversight of medical practice, as should similar allegations when they relate to events at 'conventional' rehabilitation centres. In this instance, this could be the NSW Medical Board or the Australian Medical Association.

The Brain Injury Therapy Centre's outcomes attacked

The Report's conclusions considered above attack the theoretical basis of Freeman's approach to rehabilitation, his clinical competence, the facilities available at the BITC and the practices undertaken there. Three other conclusions consist of criticisms of the value of treatment provided at the BITC. The first is that:

- The therapy provided at the Brain Injury Therapy Centre will not improve the overall degree of disability of the patients.

In the background to this conclusion, some statistics drawn from a paper by Bryan Jennett are cited. The greatest prominence among these is accorded to Jennett's statement that 95 per cent of people reach their final outcome level of recovery after brain injury by 12 months post trauma. This figure is coupled with another—namely, that most patients entered the BITC one to four years after their injury.

Referring to the patient and family stories in Chapters 2 and 3, it will be recalled that people coming to Freeman's attention, either in the BITC or elsewhere, had often been deemed unsuitable for conventional rehabilitation programs during the preceding period. Following rejection from the conventional system, placement in a nursing home or similar institution was common. Freeman had agitated, with uniform lack of success, to have his methods tested on 'early entrants' like the person cited above in the report, who had entered Coorabel Rehabilitation Hospital within weeks of her accident.

The only valid comparison group for assessing whether the BITC had benefited its patients would be people with brain injuries of similar severity who had *not* been retrieved from aged or terminal-care placements. One may assume, with considerable confidence, that no health minister would wish to bring *their* histories into the public domain.

A second of the Report's conclusions was that the treatment offered at the BITC would not assist patient rehabilitation:

- The treatment programs at the Brain Injury Therapy Centre are not regarded as effectual programs for rehabilitation of brain injury.

The information on this page is sourced to BITC 'personal communication'. It describes a number of sets of manoeuvres to be undertaken with a specific patient. This is footnoted with a comment from a leading (as usual, anonymous) rehabilitation specialist: 'As a rehabilitation program for someone four years post-trauma, I have to say that it's simply rubbish.'

The supporting information for this conclusion exemplifies the recurrent features of this Report. First, the opinions relating to Freeman's practices are of anonymous origin. Perhaps this was considered to be essential given the defamatory nature of much of the opinion? Second, the content of the Report is almost invariably based on snippets of patient information without any indication of context. Contextual background information on patient age, nature of injury and preceding patient experience in more conventional rehabilitation services is invariably lacking. Third, comparisons between the patients who had graduated into a group overseen by the anonymous leading rehabilitation specialist and Freeman's patients who had already emphatically failed that test are meaningless.

The history of this patient of Freeman's during the four years after injury would be quite revealing. One's guess is that he or she is likely to have spent most of that time, after rejection as 'unsuitable for rehabilitation', in a warehousing situation of sensory deprivation. The last two words of the leading specialist's opinion might provide a useful description of much of the Report. Who knows?

A third conclusion offered a view on strategies for rehabilitation:

- Gentle, non-intensive 'coma stimulation' programs for a limited time period are the only kind of coma arousal now practised in orthodox medical centres in the US.

This conclusion is based on opinions expressed by three US rehabilitation specialists and one Australian who had visited the United States. The content of those practitioners' comments includes one that the value of coma arousal is unproven, another that it is very difficult to measure the effectiveness of coma arousal, a third that controlled trials would be very difficult to conduct and finally a comment that coma arousal was being used by the respondent at a low intensity.

The sample size from which opinion has been sought is extremely small. Had Cuff Consultants taken the time to read the 1983 volume of the journal *Physical Therapy* discussed above, they would have been better informed. A conclusion that might equally well be drawn from the 26 lines of supporting information accompanying the conclusion is that coma arousal has not been validated and that, methodologically, it will be difficult to do so. The reference in the Report's conclusion to 'orthodox' centres could hardly be taken as something with which Freeman could disagree. His ideas for brain injury management were certainly not regarded as orthodox in Australia in the 1980s. A third Cuff Report conclusion was that:

Freeman's rehabilitation therapy will cost too much

- The therapy advocated by the Brain Injury Therapy Centre could raise the cost of third party claims.

The final section of the Report suggests that the BITC might increase the cost of third-party insurance claims. It is concluded that 'the therapy is more labour-intensive than the nursing home level of care normally given to people with an outcome of profoundly severe physical and cognitive disability'. Apart from raising the issue of relative costs of the BITC and nursing homes, the Report floats the possibility that there may not be sufficient numbers of people with profound physical and cognitive disability to fill it 'at a desirable capacity'. A concluding point raised in the Report is that the BITC does not have sufficient of the right mix of staffing.

When the Report draws attention to the differences between the BITC and what is 'normally' done in nursing homes, I can at last agree, with the proviso that 'usually' be substituted for 'normally'. One might suspect that the Report conclusion that the BITC might increase costs took account of views expressed by its commissioning personnel.

The original decision of the GIO to fund Freeman's work on behalf of people with severe brain injuries could be seen as substantially humanitarian. One might speculate that, reflecting personnel changes within the organisation, recognition dawned that humanitarian considerations come at a cost. If so, perhaps it became necessary for humanitarian considerations to become more subsidiary to financial ones. When one recalls the enthusiastic response of all participants, including the GIO, to the improvised facilities when the centre opened, the report's identification of the architectural inadequacy of the buildings—potentially, another looming expense for the GIO if the operation were to continue—is consistent with the speculation above.

Specialists implicated in preparation of the Cuff Report

The final page of the Report is headed 'Specialists'. It lists 19 individuals, five of whom are identified by name at various places in the body of the Report. It would be reasonable to infer that all of those listed had been consulted during preparation of the Report, however, it is clear that this certainly was not the case. Freeman's inquiries of two of the named specialists—Professor Sheldon Berrol, Head of Rehabilitation Medicine at the San Francisco General Hospital, and James Lance, Professor of Neurology at the University of New South Wales—determined that they had not been contacted and could not therefore have commented on the report, whilst a third, Bernard Amos, Director General of Health for New South Wales, had met Cuff but had not had any discussion about the BITC with him.

Assessing the Cuff Report

What, then is one to make of the Cuff report? It consistently fails to grasp the concept of testing evidence in a scientific manner. It could be read as an array of opinions justifying the withdrawal of funding support to the BITC. Certainly, staffing changes at the GIO around the time of commissioning the Report resulted in a change of personnel overseeing the BITC. As noted in Chapter 6, Freeman considered that the original GIO decision to fund his approach to management of brain injury was not solely a commercial decision but owed something to a genuine humanitarian concern. If so, perhaps commercial imperatives were reasserting their primacy?

Another puzzling aspect surrounding the Report is the two-year gap, almost to the day, between its presentation to the GIO and its public release by Collins in the NSW Parliament. Collins was to maintain in later years that he was doing no more than reading out advice received from his department. This does not explain why the Report was withheld from the public for two years. Assuming the GIO accepted the findings of the Report in March 1987, it could be convincingly argued that it was deficient in its disbursement of public money in permitting funding of the BITC to proceed for another two years after this. On the other hand, if the GIO found the Report not to be credible, it might have been expected to file it away permanently and allow the moths to have their way, not to release it to the minister when a GIO executive deemed this to be appropriate. One might speculate that the release of the Report was a made-to-order circuit-breaker to afford an opportunity for curtailment of expenditure.

Two opinions of the Cuff Report's overall scientific veracity might be cited at this point. A neuropsychologist from a major university wrote concerning the Cuff Report:

> [T]his report will have to be judged of such appalling standard as to be deemed a parody of professional commentary. I sincerely hope it has never influenced anyone's decision making as such could only be a basis for travesty. The author provides us with no definitions, terms of reference, description of methodology, list of working assumptions, account of his own qualifications or operational model for the evaluation of a therapeutic process. Without these conventional niceties the report is fairly viewed as a political document likely to introduce unspecified biases and proceed by exacerbating existing controversy. This particular report is rather worse than that as it purports to introduce relevant evidence. In so doing the author displays gross ignorance on every technical issue raised and a willingness to construct evidence in such a way that it constitutes a deliberate process of deceit.

It is also my view that before a neutral tribunal a very strong case can be made that any administrative decisions and their consequences based on this report were either based on misadvice or irresponsibly taken. If anyone has been foolish enough to take this report seriously I can see many good grounds for having it exposed to judicial scrutiny. After all Mr Cuff has made a vicious attack on an important practitioner working in an area inevitably steeped in human misery.[10]

Another reviewer, an educational psychologist, wrote:

I have examined the 'Report of the Brain Injury Division' prepared by Cuff and Associates (March 1987) and have reached the conclusion that this document can in no way be described as a research report.

Summary: This report which roundly criticises Dr Freeman for his lack of research basis, is itself totally without a solid research basis ... Its conclusions concerning both the operations of the Brain Injury Therapy Centre and its medical director, Dr Ted Freeman, are in no way justified on the basis of the very slim evidence put forward in this report.[11]

In the aftermath of the incorporation of the Report into parliamentary proceedings, Freeman has expressed his opinions on the issue of parliamentary privilege as follows:

There are three basic components.

First, every Member of Parliament must act with integrity and ensure that his or her statements are based on knowledge that is honest and accurate.

Second, any person whose reputation is likely to suffer from adverse comments to be made under parliamentary privilege should be made aware of the charges against him or her and be given the opportunity to refute them before they are raised in Parliament.

Third, a mechanism should exist which allows redress in Parliament for incorrect and misleading statements made under parliamentary privilege.

In relation to the minister's speech, he considered, very reasonably:

Collins had made a series of critical thrusts at me and virtually called me an impostor taking advantage of 'helpless people unprotected by any legislation'.

---

10 John Masters, Letter to Freeman, 13 June 1990.
11 Cecile Ferguson, Letter to Freeman, June 1990.

Collins had used a document in the House without ensuring its accuracy. This had done enormous damage to people with severe brain injury and to my work and had blocked a new approach to therapy for some of the most disadvantaged people in the country.

Freeman, and others acting on his behalf, attempted over the course of the decade following Collins' statement to obtain redress in the NSW Parliament. He has described one approach:

I found that there was a mechanism known as a Citizen's Right of Reply. I wrote to the Speaker of the Legislative Assembly seeking such a right. I referred to Collins' comments and wrote—

The comments were detrimental to my pioneering work with those who have been severely brain injured. I have adequate medical support from Australian and international sources to refute the claims made.

The Speaker replied: 'Unfortunately, as the proceedings you refer to predate the passage of the Legislative Assembly's resolution on 26th November 1996, regarding a citizen's right of reply, I am unable to consider your request.'

The events that ultimately led the NSW Legislative Assembly to have a correction introduced into *Hansard* were a reflection of the high regard in which Ted Freeman was held by his colleagues, both in Australia and overseas. As such, they can most appropriately be told in the context of medical support for him, which is the subject of the following chapter. Before concluding this account, however, it would be timely to give an indication of the manner in which the Cuff Report and its uncritical promulgation by Collins was to be used to inflict further damage on Freeman.

One of the occasions on which Freeman was denied access to a hospital when families had asked him to assess their inpatient relative occurred in April 1995. In this instance, the ACT Director of Rehabilitation Services had requested the hospital administration to ensure his exclusion. In response to this, Freeman and two friends—a retired ACT Supreme Court judge and myself—found ourselves sitting in the hospital boardroom facing three others: the rehabilitation director, the clinical superintendent and the dean of the local medical school.

It became abundantly clear as the meeting became increasingly combative that the patients' families were not going to have their wishes fulfilled. The *pièce de résistance* came when the dean, in a superbly choreographed performance, read the Collins statement in its entirety as the definitive reason Freeman was not wanted in that hospital.

Parenthetically, it could be noted that the preceding anecdote related to the hospital at which Freeman's exclusion resulted in his examination of Louise in the hospital car park (see above). Some years later, during a burst of media interest in brain injury, the National Brain Injury Foundation was contacted to ascertain whether a patient who had improved following a very poor prognosis could be located in time for the evening program. Louise immediately came to mind. Unfortunately, the opportunity to secure some viewing time for brain injury was lost. She was competing in track and field at the Athens Paralympics. As a postscript, it can be added that, at the time of writing, she has this week won a silver medal in the shot-put at the London Paralympics.

Conclusion

A number of reasons for the strong opposition directed at Ted Freeman and his clinical practices were advanced during the 1980s and 1990s. For instance, the claims by patients' families, and in some instances, by the patients themselves, that very worthwhile improvement had occurred during the course of a Freeman program were often flatly contradictory of pessimistic prognoses issued by acute-care practitioners. Similarly, when Freeman espoused community-based domiciliary rehabilitation, he was challenging the prerogative of several groups of medical and paramedical practitioners to make all rehabilitation decisions.

Whilst the above reasons are likely to have loomed large in fuelling opposition, the reason most commonly advanced was probably that Freeman had not presented any scientifically validated data to support his contention that active attempts at stimulation would be of more benefit for people remaining unconscious following brain injury than the established practice of 'wait and see'. The irony of this reasoning was that the 'wait and see' approach was itself totally lacking in any scientific validation. The precept underlying it—namely, that the damaged mammalian brain heals better if sensory input is minimised— was longstanding but remained no more than unproven theory.

Although independent scientific evidence supporting the theoretical basis for Freeman's propositions was unavailable at the time when he was putting them into practice, more recent discoveries have provided some strong support. The ongoing refinement of techniques for scanning the human brain in order to detect activity that cannot be observed by clinical observation has yielded new insights relevant to Freeman's clinical management strategies. For example, it has been established that stimuli with strong personal relevance, such as speaking the patient's name, are consistently recognised by some brain injured people, notwithstanding the absence of any response that is clinically apparent. Another observation has been that responses to stimuli during the early stages of awakening from coma may occur only intermittently, a phenomenon originally characterised by Freeman as 'soft signs'.

One of the outcomes of increasing recognition that Freeman's proposals represented an advance on the prevailing attitude towards rehabilitation after brain injury has been their gradual incorporation into the practice of others. Whilst that incorporation has not usually been accompanied by acknowledgment, there have been some notable exceptions. One of these, provided by neurosurgeon Professor Donald Simpson and already cited above, merits repetition: 'Freeman's work has stimulated an overall improvement in rehabilitation services and he has played a respectable role in the development of rehabilitation in Australia.' This appraisal was provided shortly after the 1989 attack in the NSW Parliament and was a response to that attack.

Paradoxically, although Freeman was criticised for not providing firm evidence of the efficacy of his approach, some of his critics who were well placed and resourced to document the results of the conventional approach had failed to make any attempt to do so. I refer to the BIRP units discussed above, which were unable to provide historical information on the outcomes of rehabilitation programs undertaken with brain injured people.

A few general implications of the responses encountered by Freeman are worth noting. Caution about adopting novel therapeutic responses to any medical condition is quite justifiable. The same cannot be said of the mind-set underpinning the opposition, ranging from the petty to the highly destructive, which Freeman experienced. When a practitioner is not prepared to discuss alternative approaches to the treatment of a patient's condition with a fellow practitioner who is advocating change, that refusal says more about the first practitioner than about the colleague. The complete divergence between Australian and leading international practitioners in their appraisal of any form of therapy is both puzzling and disconcerting. It is not necessary that Australian practitioners follow overseas practice without question. It is necessary, surely, that they be aware of differences between practices. Especially disappointing in this context was the inability of the NHMRC, even as late as 1995, to think again about revisiting an earlier pronouncement.

Finally, and of very general significance, Freeman's case adds to a considerable existing body of legitimate concern about parliamentary privilege. When ministers and those supporting them fail to exercise responsibility before issuing statements that are likely to damage others, often irreversibly once the media disseminates them, that represents a blatant abuse of privilege.

8. International support forthcoming

If one is to attempt to form an unbiased assessment of the value of Freeman's work, it is clearly necessary to search beyond the hostile opinions some examples of which were given in the preceding chapter. One possible approach would be to examine the extent to which his proposals for management of people with severe brain injuries have been reflected in clinical practice during the three decades since he began to apply them. Another, more direct, course of action could be to refer to evaluations of the man and his work by others with acknowledged expertise in this field. Both will be considered below.

When seeking to assess the value of a clinician's practices by determining the extent to which the direction of the practice of others subsequently came to resemble them, it is essential to recognise that, with rare exceptions, the evolution of clinical practice and the thinking underlying it are likely to reflect a succession of contributions from many clinicians. That said, the temporal sequence of modifications in practice may be quite informative. If, for instance, advocacy by a clinician of a practice that is not generally accepted is followed, some time later, by the acceptance of that practice as legitimate in 'mainstream' medicine, it is possible that the original advocacy has contributed to its acceptance. In its simplest form, such a contribution might be affirmed by its acknowledgment as a citation in the literature.

If modifications of attitudes and resulting practices have occurred through a gradual series of changes, this is likely to militate against direct linkage of contemporary practice to proposals advanced from a single source several decades earlier. It may not be justified to infer that, because more generalised adoption of a particular approach to therapy followed some time after earlier advocacy for it, that advocacy had caused the adoption. Nevertheless, that adoption certainly supports the value of the modifications that formed the basis of the preceding advocacy

Taking account of the inevitable limitations to tracing the origin of changes in clinical practice, it is informative to scan the published literature on coma arousal over the 30 years since Freeman's original advocacy for change. At the outset, it is extremely likely that Freeman's ideas, although independently derived, would have been strongly influenced by those of US clinicians responsible for the operation of highly specialised rehabilitation clinics such as that of Danese Malkmus outlined in Chapter 4.

International research and practice

A 1994 paper from an Ohio medical centre in the *Journal of Neurosurgical Nursing*, rather provocatively titled 'Early intervention: coma stimulation in the intensive care ward', presented the case for a greatly expanded role for coma arousal at an earlier time after injury. The ideas presented in this paper could have passed as a summary of Freeman's hopes at the time of the 'Westmead' trial described in an earlier chapter. The abstract merits quoting in full:

> Coma stimulation is a technique that has traditionally been reserved for patients in a rehabilitation setting. Information regarding the use of coma stimulation in the intensive care setting is limited. An individualized coma stimulation program in the early stages of recovery from brain injury is paramount in stimulating the reticular activating system and promoting brain reorganization. Coma stimulation program development within the intensive care setting includes the appropriate selection of patients and the utilization of the entire rehabilitation team in devising an approach specific to each patient's needs. Planning should include the family, with consideration given to the prior interests of the patient. Ongoing evaluation of the patient's responses should be considered as well as the ease of performing stimulation within the intensive care environment.[1]

Freeman advocated the early implementation of arousal programs but, while a few families undertook these informally in intensive care wards, most of his patients had sustained their injuries months, if not years, before attempts at stimulation. The emphasis on family involvement in stimulation and on exploiting a patient's prior interests in this 1994 paper accord precisely with Freeman's aspirations.

Whilst the 2009 Cochrane review of publications on coma arousal to which reference was made in Chapter 6 covered the period 1996–2002, the paper of Sosnowski and Ustik from Ohio noted above, not being a clinical trial, was not considered in it. All of the publications to be cited below, which reported trials, fell outside the period covered by the review.

In 2003, another article published in the same journal, in this instance from the University of Michigan School of Nursing, reported on a small 'quasi-experimental' study undertaken in an intensive care setting. A group of 12 patients was introduced into a 'structured auditory sensory stimulation program' three days after injury and this was continued for seven days. The outcome

---

1   Cheryl Sosnowski & Melissa Ustik (1994) Early intervention: coma stimulation in the intensive care unit. *Journal of Neuroscience Nursing*, 26, 336.

in this small group suggested that the program may have promoted arousal. Perhaps more importantly, taking account of criticism of Freeman on the basis of potential harmful effects of stimulation, no adverse effects on parameters of patients' brain status were observed notwithstanding the very early stage of this intervention.[2]

Also in 2003, two members of the Faculty of Nursing at the University of Calgary published an article described as 'a conceptual analysis', which discusses the comparative merits of coma arousal, based on the provision of high degrees of stimulation and a 'sensory regulation' approach. The latter was described as comprising 'information processing and mediation of reaction to sensory information with emphasis on enhancing selective attention by regulating the environment'. Aside from the comparison, it was noted that both approaches have in common

> the belief that the person in a persistent vegetative state may, at some level, be able to perceive and begin to process information and that external stimulation may enhance that process. Nurses interacting with persons in persistent vegetative state are encouraged to think about how they can regulate sensory input to enhance meaning and facilitate information processing for these patients.[3]

In 2004, another report, in this instance from the Shanghai Second Medical University, examined 175 patients who had been comatose for periods of at least one month. The arousal procedures that were tested included exposure to hyperbaric oxygen, physical therapy and arousal drugs. The frequency of regaining consciousness decreased with the length of the period in coma. Nevertheless, the authors concluded that 'the application of appropriate arousal procedures improves recovery of consciousness in patients with prolonged coma'.[4]

A review from the intensive care unit of a San Diego hospital published in *Critical Care Nursing Quarterly* in 2005 canvassed the question of the adequacy of existing management of comatose patients in the following terms:

> Today, healthcare professionals are being encouraged to research and explore the possibility of implementing structured coma stimulation programs as early as 72 hours postinjury in the intensive care unit.

---

2   Alice E. Davis & Ana Gimenez (2003) Cognitive-behavioral recovery in comatose patients following auditory sensory stimulation. *Journal of Neuroscience Nursing, 35,* 202.
3   Patrizia Tolle & Marlene Reimer (2003) Do we need stimulation programs as a part of nursing care for patients in 'persistent vegetative state'? A conceptual analysis. *Axone, 25,* 20.
4   Jy Jiang, Y. H. Bo, Y. H. Yin, Y. H. Pan, Y. M. Liang & Q. Z. Luo (2004) Effect of arousal methods for 175 cases of prolonged coma after severe traumatic brain injury and its related factors. *Chinese Journal of Traumatology, 7,* 341–3.

Starting early is of paramount importance to a patient's survival, quality of life and overall long-term prognosis. The goal of this article is to educate healthcare professionals (in the hospital setting) about managing and implementing structured sensory stimulation sessions.[5]

A 2010 Chinese report of attempts to arouse comatose patients utilised an approach reflecting its source. The aim of this study was '[t]o observe the therapeutic effect of continuous electroacupuncture for arousing consciousness of comatose patients with severe craniocerebral trauma'. An interesting reflection on the investigators' perspective was their description of the control group as receiving 'traditional western medicine'—namely, nothing more than nursing care. Of 56 entering subjects, all with a Glasgow Coma Scale score lower than 8, half were randomly selected into the acupuncture group. The arousal rate after both one and three months was significantly higher in the group receiving the experimental treatment.[6]

Whether any of the preceding reports owed something to Freeman's publications cannot be determined. What they do demonstrate is that ideas very similar to those espoused by him in the 1980s have been expressed in the 2000s by healthcare professionals working in high-quality facilities. The implementation of arousal programs in an intensive care ward was something to which he had aspired but which had never been possible in the environment within which he was working. All of these papers expressed the premise that patients remaining in coma might have retained some level of awareness without the capacity to indicate this to others. Notable similarities between the approaches described in these reports and that of Freeman, apart from the repeated advocacy and practice of very early intervention, included the importance of family involvement and the value of introducing environmental cues with which patients had been familiar before brain injury. The leading role envisaged for nurses, rather than medical practitioners, evidenced in the authorship of these reports, is also strongly in accord with his beliefs.

The methods suggested to facilitate arousal varied with the institution—strategies varied between structured stimulation and sensory regulation—reflecting local practices, for example, the use of acupuncture in one of the Chinese studies. The description cited above, by Chinese authors, of the 'non-intervention' approach as 'traditional western medicine' provokes reflection on its scientific origins (or on the lack thereof).

---

5   Carolyn S. Gerber (2005) Understanding and managing coma stimulation: are we doing everything we can? *Critical Care Nursing Quarterly, 28*, 94.
6   Fan Peng, Ze-qi Chen & Jie-kun Luo (2010) Clinical observation on continuous electroacupuncture at Neiguan (PC 6) for arousing consciousness of comatose patients with severe craniocerebral trauma. *Zhongguo Zhen Jiu [Chinese Acupuncture and Moxibustion], 30*, 465.

None of the reports cited above was contributed by Australian sources. A search of the US National Institutes of Health 'PubMed' web site failed to uncover any Australian papers either promoting or rejecting coma arousal procedures apart from Freeman's publications and one paper from a Westmead Hospital group relating to the abandoned trial. Freeman published a response to this report in the same journal. The absence of local publications with relevance to coma arousal is not particularly informative as, in the absence of novel information, there may be little impetus for practitioners to publish or for editors to accede to that impetus. That said, it hardly suggests the existence of a vigorous culture of research among Australian rehabilitation practitioners.

Evolution of Australian practice in management of prolonged coma

Finding documentation of Australian management practice of people who remain unconscious following brain injury is difficult given the apparent absence of any publications in peer-reviewed journals. One interesting exception has been provided by the minutes of a meeting between the Board of the National Brain Injury Foundation and a rehabilitation specialist from the University of Sydney, Professor Denis Smith. This meeting occurred on 11 June 1993 at the Royal Rehabilitation Centre, Ryde. Denis Smith is reported as saying that '[t]here is now a belief that many of the things Dr Freeman has been saying over the years are true, that is, if you stimulate people at a critical time in their recovery, the prognosis might well be better'.

The minutes continue:

> Professor Smith went on to say that institutional services need to be far better than they are, and it is important that they learn from Dr Freeman and others the nature and best type of service that should be provided to people in the community. He added the reason he attended the meeting was that he believes that for a significant number of people Dr Freeman's program is better than the alternative.

> Professor Smith stated that Dr Freeman looks after people from his (Smith's) unit who it was felt would be better treated at home. They are not (officially) referred to Dr Freeman but rather are told, 'You can go and see Dr Freeman'.

In contrast with the negative Australian responses to Freeman's ideas and practice, expressed in several ways, which were recounted in the preceding chapter, he received strongly positive assessments from leading clinicians in the

United States and United Kingdom over an extended period. This took the form of unreserved approbation of his monograph *The Catastrophe of Coma*, and of refinements to practice that he pioneered, most notably his Coma Exit Chart.

Appreciation of his achievements also took the form of invitations to small group meetings of leading international practitioners in the field of brain injury. This contrasted with his simultaneous Australian experience of exclusion from participation in meetings of rehabilitation practitioners for the reason, repeatedly given, that others would not participate if he were to be invited. This contrast in assessment of Freeman's work raises questions about some aspects of Australian medical practice that should be concerning. These are briefly examined in the conclusion to Chapter 7. Finally, and most emphatically, his international standing was unequivocally affirmed by letters of support in response to his efforts to have his reputation reinstated in Australia after it was besmirched under parliamentary privilege. These letters are considered below.

International appraisal of Freeman's publications

It will be recalled from the preceding chapter that the attack on Freeman in the NSW Legislative Assembly, which effectively destroyed his efforts to assist people who had not been helped by traditional rehabilitation methods, occurred in 1989. The Australian edition of his first book, *The Catastrophe of Coma*, was published in 1987. The US edition was published in 1989. Responses to it from clinicians who were, arguably, much better qualified to assess rehabilitation after brain injury than any contemporary Australian rehabilitation practitioners provide stark contrasts with the frequently anonymous opinions cited in the Cuff Report.

For example, the foreword to the US edition of *The Catastrophe of Coma* was contributed by Professor Henry Stonnington, Director of the Research and Training Center for the Severely Head Injured at the Medical College of Virginia, Virginia Commonwealth University, Richmond, and Professor of Rehabilitation Medicine at the university. Stonnington was also the Editor-in-Chief of the international journal *Brain Injury*. He wrote:

> Dr Ted Freeman is a pioneer. Like many pioneers he does what he thinks is right. He knows that coma patients can improve when handled in certain ways. He has confidence that something can be done in many cases. He has devised a coma care delivery system which relies heavily on family involvement. Who better to help the victim than the family?

The book is not only a must for all the families and friends of brain injury victims but also for the professionals who treat them. Here we have a method of management which is not only sound—even if not proved scientifically—but also one which is fiscally responsible and can be afforded by everyone whether living in a large town or a small rural community.

Congratulations to Dr Freeman for his innovative approach and for all the hope he gives to victims, friends and families.

A number of points raised in this foreword merit emphasis. Apart from his very positive endorsement of Freeman's strategy of working through the agency of the family, Stonnington suggests that the book will be a 'must' for rehabilitation clinicians. Contrast this with the apparently organised attacks on Freeman by a section of the Australian rehabilitation profession, specialty groups such as the Australian Association of Neurologists and a national regulatory body, the NHMRC. Stonnington has explicitly made the point that the absence of 'scientific' proof of a method that has been shown to be clinically sound should not preclude its adoption.

Reflecting on the events surrounding the abortive Westmead trial described in Chapter 6, it would not be unduly difficult to interpret the abandonment of a trial as more of an excuse than a reason for resistance to Freeman's approach. Finally, Stonnington has credited the strategy described in the book with being 'fiscally responsible'. This contrasts with the condemnation of Freeman's approach in the Cuff Report on the grounds of its inferred expense.

A transatlantic appreciation of *The Catastrophe of Coma*, also written in 1989, was provided by Dr Keith Andrews, the Director of Medical and Research Services at the Royal Hospital for Neurodisability in London. He considered:

> It is extremely good though to be quite honest I would be very frightened to give it to relatives of patients in my Unit until after they have left us. To have the relatives pressuring us even more to fit in with your recommendations would I think result in closure of the Unit.[7]

Another strong English endorsement of Freeman's work was provided by Dr Clarke of the British Life Insurance Trust for Health Education:

> *The Catastrophe of Coma—a Way Back*, is a really excellent book and I would like to congratulate everyone involved in its production. We have been raising money to distribute free of charge Coma Stimulation Kits to hospitals. What I would like to do is include the book with the kit.[8]

---

7   Keith Andrews, Letter to Freeman, 20 March 1989.
8   Donald Clarke, Letter to Michael White, 20 July 1988.

Some time after publication of this book, Freeman met Professor George Zitnay, the President of the International Brain Injury Association and the CEO of the US National Head Injury Foundation. He recalls:

> *He congratulated me on my book,* The Catastrophe of Coma—a Way Back. *I asked, 'Would the US National Head Injury Foundation be interested in publishing another edition of my book, as it is now out of print?' 'Yes,' he replied, 'we would be pleased to consider such a proposition.' I then showed him the draft of my new book,* Brain Injury and Stroke—a Handbook to Recovery, *which recorded my recommendations on the rehabilitation of people with a severe brain injury in their own home. 'Would you be interested in publishing this book as well?' I asked. He replied, 'Yes, we may be interested. Could you let me have a copy?' I was very pleased.*

Freeman received a letter from the National Head Injury Foundation:

> I would like to inform you that the National Head Injury Foundation [NHIF] endorses your publications: *The Catastrophe of Coma—a Way Back* (1987) and *Brain Injury and Stroke—a Handbook to Recovery* (1995). Indeed we would be pleased to be involved in the publication and dissemination of these remarkable books. We at the NHIF applaud and admire your courageous approach to the cause of individuals with TBI [traumatic brain injury] and wish you all the best in your endeavour to champion this noble cause.[9]

But things did not work out that way. In early 1996, Professor George Zitnay wrote that the legal advisors to the US National Head Injury Association had said that the publication of Freeman's books would jeopardise their non-profit status. Professor Zitnay wrote: 'I regret we are unable to act as publishers. However, the National Head Injury Association would be willing to assist in promoting the book and disseminate it through our Catalogue of Educational Materials.'

The preceding assessments refer to Freeman's achievement in devising his approach to coma management, in applying his ideas in a clinical setting and in presenting them in a form intended for, and accessible to, both families and professionals. In the decade following the publication of his second book, the author conducted what was effectively a mobile solo practice, travelling, as described in Chapter 7, to patients' homes. Nevertheless, the development, refining and testing of his ideas continued. Reference has already been made to his earlier attempts to meet a major need—namely, that of documenting the pace of emergence from coma. This was sometimes slow and irregular and could only be observed inconsistently in its early stages.

---

9   National Head Injury Foundation, Letter to Freeman, 17 April 1995.

International acceptance and adoption of the Coma Exit Chart

A second major achievement, resulting from his years of working with patients and their families, was Freeman's introduction of the Coma Exit Chart, described in Chapter 4. As should be evident from reading the stories of patients and their families in earlier chapters, that emergence from coma, although it tends to be well publicised when it occurs abruptly after a prolonged period of coma, can be much more difficult to detect.

Signs of awakening and awareness may be accessible to eliciting and observable at one time of day but not at another. They may be entirely dependent on individually specific circumstances such as the identity of person(s) attempting to elicit a response and objects or sounds peculiar to the individual. Whilst often difficult to document, especially in the early stages, a patient's responses can be a critical guide to further management and prognosis.

Freeman's description of his Coma Exit Chart was first published in the journal *Brain Injury* in 1996. It has impacted substantially upon the management of comatose patients in some leading overseas clinics. Other charts in use overseas have been based on Freeman's original, not invariably with appropriate attribution.

Two appraisals of Freeman's contribution to detecting awakening were also cited in Chapter 4. To summarise their content, Dr Sarah Wilson, senior lecturer in the Department of Psychological Medicine in the University of Glasgow, indicated that she routinely used the chart and that she considered Freeman's work had generated further research internationally. Keith Andrews of the Royal Hospital for Neurodisability in London considered that Freeman's exit chart filled a primary role in the standard UK procedure for assessment of emergence from coma.

In attempting to assign a level of significance to any piece of research, the opinions of well-qualified and independent peers are invaluable. Perhaps even more important are indications of the extent to which the research under consideration has resulted in changing the thinking, practice or research of the persons responding to requests for an assessment.

The assessments of Wilson and Andrews imply that, at least in the United Kingdom, Freeman's Coma Exit Chart had exerted a major influence on clinical practice. Parenthetically, the date of publication of the first paper in *Brain Injury* describing the chart was 1996. This might be placed alongside the opinions being promulgated at that time in Australia about Freeman—for example, the official opinion of the NHMRC. Reference to the preceding chapter will again disclose considerable discrepancy between the 'home' and the international scenes.

Invitations to present Freeman's research at international conferences

Another yardstick of the extent to which any researcher's contribution is valued by his or her peers is the occurrence of invitations to contribute to the formulation of 'high-level' recommendations. It will be recalled that Freeman was most emphatically blackballed from several Australian meetings (not especially 'high powered') intended to explore possibilities for research into management of coma. The grounds given for exclusion to those endeavouring to ensure his participation were that, if he was included in the program, other potential participants would withdraw.

Taking note of events in Australia, it may come as a surprise that Freeman was invited to some small group meetings overseas at which the other participants would undoubtedly qualify for description as international leaders in the field. A most significant year for Ted Freeman was 1989, as it was for the implementation of his ideas on management of coma, with the attack on both in the NSW Legislative Assembly on 1 March. Again, the contrast between local and international perceptions of his work came into sharp focus.

He was invited by the International Association for the Study of Traumatic Brain Injury (IASTBI) to present a medical paper on coma arousal therapy at the First World Conference on Traumatic Brain Injury, which was held in San Jose, California, in April 1989. Freeman has summarised his impression of this conference:

> It was a relief to be amongst professionals who were seeking ways to improve the care of those who had suffered brain injury. It was also fascinating that while the medical profession had been slow to come to grips with this problem in the United States, the neuropsychologists and psychologists had become interested and were forcing the pace of reform.

In September of the same year, Freeman presented a paper on coma arousal therapy at the International Conference on Brain Injury in London. In the course of discussions with clinicians and researchers from half a dozen countries, a proposal evolved for a multinational research study on coma. The study was envisaged as a collaborative project jointly based in Glasgow, London and Sydney. Taking account of the events in Sydney during 1989, what followed became predictable. Freeman recalls:

> Some months after the conference in London, Dr Woods wrote to me asking 'to know urgently whether you wish to take part in the collaborative study'. I replied that the Brain Injury Therapy Centre could not take part in the study because, following the devastating repercussions of the Cuff Report, I knew that no government support or funding would be available to enable the therapy centre to participate in this groundbreaking venture.

Interest in the possibility of some level of recovery in patients who remained comatose in the longer term continued to increase among clinicians in a number of overseas clinics that specialised in their management. In 1991, Andrews reported in the *British Medical Journal* that 15 per cent of patients in the Royal Hospital for Neurodisability who had been diagnosed as remaining comatose six months after brain injury had subsequently improved significantly.[10] In response to this observation, he set about gathering participants for an international working party on the persistent vegetative state (PVS). This resulted in the mounting of a meeting, 'PVS 95', in London in 1995.

The goal of PVS 95 was spelled out in an article in *Brain Injury*, which reported on its outcomes:

> The need for a Working Party on the Management of the Vegetative State was identified when several specialists in neurorehabilitation expressed concern that there were no formal guidelines for the treatment of patients in the vegetative state. There had been several working parties which discussed the ethical issues, but none which had discussed the management of patients, which it was felt was required before ethical decisions such as withdrawal of tube-feeding or resource allocation could be made.[11]

Participants in PVS 95 were invited from the United Kingdom, the United States, Germany, Sweden, Israel, France, Russia, Japan and Australia. The aim of the meeting was to think beyond the prevailing established beliefs about the nature and outcomes of PVS. Freeman was the only invitee from Australia in a highly selective list of those regarded as being at the cutting edge. The extent of selection may be best conveyed by listing the names and geographical spread of the participants, as listed in Andrews' report of the meeting in *Brain Injury* in 1996.

---

10   Keith Andrews (1991) Persistent vegetative state. *British Medical Journal, 303*, 121.
11   Keith Andrews (1996) International working party on the management of the vegetative state. *Brain Injury, 11*, 797.

The working party consisted of specialists in neurological rehabilitation, neurosurgeons, neurologists and neuropsychologists from around the world. They were Dr Keith Andrews (Chairman, UK); Professor Graham Beaumont (UK); Dr Francois Danze (France); Dr Mihai D. Dimancescu (USA); Professor Axel Fugl-Meyer (Sweden); Dr E. Freeman (Australia): Dr Zeev Groswasser (Israel); Professor Bryan Jennett (UK); Dr James Kelly (USA); Professor Jean Francois Mathe (France); Professor Alexander Potapov (Russia); Dr Jay Rosenberg (USA); Professor Dr Med. Paull-Walter Schonle (Germany); Dr Henry H. Stonnington (USA); Dr Francois Tasseau (France); Professor T. Tsubokawa (Japan); Dr Sarah L. Wilson (UK); Dr Roger L. Wood (UK); Dr Nathan D. Zasler (USA); Dr George A. Zitnay (USA).

Freeman summarised his impressions of this meeting:

It was a bit daunting to have the responsibility of presenting a medical paper to such an international and distinguished group of people in the august precincts of the Royal College of Physicians. When the time came to give my paper, I walked to the front of the lecture theatre and stood while Lord Walton introduced me.

My paper was concerned with the care of so-called vegetative patients in their own homes. This was a very difficult subject because most of the patients whom I had been asked to assess over the years had been diagnosed as vegetative but were in fact locked in. Therefore I modified my paper in order to provide the hierarchical basis for the regaining of awareness and function, stressing the importance of the family in both diagnosis and treatment.

The introduction to the conference manual contained brief summaries of the background of each participant, written by Keith Andrews. In summarising Ted Freeman's achievements, he wrote:

Dr Freeman has an international reputation for his practical approach to the rehabilitation and long term management of patients in Persistent Vegetative State which is explained in his book, *The Catastrophe of Coma*. He has a particular interest in managing patients in the community and using family and non professional carers to encourage optimal levels of care.

Correcting the parliamentary record

Freeman made a number of attempts during the 1990s to have Collins' attack on him formally refuted in the NSW Legislative Assembly. In the course of attempting to rehabilitate his reputation, a number of letters from overseas specialists attesting to Freeman's professional standing were collected, and extracts from some of these were included in the parliamentary statement below. One not included, but very informative, was provided in a 2002 letter to Freeman from Ross Harris, formerly Professor of Pain Rehabilitation in the Flinders University Faculty of Medicine. Its concluding paragraph merits unabridged quotation:

> In 1999 I visited the University of Glasgow at the invitation of Sir Michael Bond, to meet with members of his brain injury research group—arguably the most impressive body of brain injury researchers in the world. My purpose was to establish collaborative links to support and strengthen our Australian longitudinal research study. At my first meeting with two professors of the University's medical faculty the discussion was all but taken over and dominated by questions from them of me about Dr Ted Freeman and his work in Sydney and Canberra. The statement was made directly to me that Dr Freeman's writings have become much valued in UK brain injury rehabilitation. Furthermore, I was informed that the senior researchers present regard you [Freeman] as one of the most interesting and important contributors to the world medical literature in brain injury rehabilitation.[12]

In accomplishing redress for disparaging statements made under privilege, a possible alternative to the unavailable Citizen's Right of Reply was to request a member of the NSW Parliament to make a statement, and Freeman succeeded in doing this. The *Hansard* records of the NSW Legislative Council, dated 2 December 2002, state that the Hon. Tony Kelly, the Deputy President of the Council, said:

> On 1 March 1989 the then Health Minister, the Hon. Peter Collins stated in another place that:

> Dr. Freeman is not conducting his work within any research framework. He does not even try to respond to requests for justification of his concepts and beliefs: he seems totally unconcerned about the rightness and wrongness of his ideas.

> The Hon. Peter Collins was understandably reliant upon advice from his advisers, who in turn relied upon a report prepared by management— not medical—consultants. That report is known as the Cuff Report.

> I am now pleased to be able to correct the views expressed by the Hon. Peter Collins in 1989 with respect to Dr. Ted Freeman. Some years ago Dr

---

12 Ross Harris, Letter to Freeman, 16 April 2002.

Freeman's son, Matthew, died as a result of a brain injury sustained in a motor accident. Shortly before this Dr Freeman had become interested in the longer term rehabilitation of people with brain injuries, and it became his mission in life until his retirement some years ago.

By walking the same path as the families of people with acquired brain injury, Dr Freeman gained insights which few of his professional colleagues shared and which, sadly, some of them dismissed as irrelevant.

Dr Freeman's internationally recognised approach to assisting patients with brain injuries and their families became known as community-based rehabilitation. It entailed learning from his patients in the very best tradition of 'pre-technological medicine' and distilling from his learning a compassionate wisdom which was to offer hope to many amid a barren mindset of therapeutic nihilism. Dr Freeman achieved a rare combination of humanitarian and cost-effective outcomes with his patients.

The reality and extent of Dr Freeman's achievement in pioneering a new response to brain injury can be best appreciated by noting assessments from two disparate sources: patients' families and international authorities on rehabilitation after brain injury. A request made in the mid-1990s by the then MHR for Gilmore, who had taken a strong interest in the subject of brain injury, was answered with scores of letters from the families of people whom Ted had helped. Any medical practitioner would have been honoured to receive testimonials such as these.

This pioneering work on brain injury therapy and intense rehabilitation was recognised recently by Justice Barry O'Keefe in a case in the Supreme Court of NSW—*Northbridge v Central Sydney Area Health Service*—in which Dr Freeman was called as an expert witness.

Justice O'Keefe acknowledged the value of seeking the views and opinions of the family of a person suffering brain injury. In closing I will cite a few recent assessments of Freeman's calibre and of his contributions.

I am writing to express my deepest appreciation to you for your outstanding work in the field of Brain Injury Recovery and Rehabilitation. You have contributed much to families of persons with brain injury (George A Zitnay, Chairman of the World Health Organization, President Emeritus of the International Brain Injury Foundation and formerly President of the Head Injury Association of America).

Dr Freeman has an international status for his work with patients and families who have been affected by the trauma of such profound brain damage (Keith Andrews, Director of Medical and Research Services, Royal Hospital for Neuro-disability, London).

Dr Freeman is recognised internationally for his expertise … His work has generated further research and is undoubtedly of benefit to patients with severe brain injury (Sarah Wilson, Senior Lecturer in Psychological Medicine, the University of Glasgow).

Dr Freeman's concept of working with brain injury victims and their families early as well as later, when others have given up, is something we all need to follow (Henry Stonington [sic], Founding Editor of the journal *Brain Injury* and retired Professor and Chair, Departments of Physical Medicine and Rehabilitation, Virginia Commonwealth University).

Ted Freeman had at last been able to clear his name.

Conclusion

In summing up this chapter, its striking feature is undoubtedly the contrast it presents if compared with the preceding one. Three differences in content stand out. The first of these concerns the attitudes expressed towards Freeman and his work. The differences could hardly be sharper: in one case, unremittingly denigrating, in the other, universally laudatory. The second difference is in the source of the expressed attitudes. Denigration originated exclusively within Australia; acclamation for his work came predominantly from overseas practitioners. The third salient difference relates to the professional standing of the practitioners assessing Freeman. Those providing strongly positive assessments were invariably pre-eminent, as judged by the positions they held in first-class institutions and also by their publication records. Those responsible for negative assessments could not be classed as pre-eminent on either count. A useful indication of the esteem in which Freeman was held by overseas practitioners is provided by reading the list of invited participants at the PVS 95 meeting described above.

Two reasons were given for attacking Freeman and disparaging his work. The theoretical basis he presented for his clinical approach was not underpinned by laboratory findings. There was consistent reluctance to accept his reports of favourable clinical outcomes attributable to his therapeutic initiatives, a reluctance that was preserved by a resistance to dialogue with the man in any scientific forum. Two responses to these two reasons should have been evident immediately they were advanced. Laboratory findings supporting the prevailing, very conservative approach to management of comatose patients were non-existent. Favourable outcomes of that conservative approach were attributed to 'natural healing', rather than to any therapy per se, hence the attitude prevailing among most Australian rehabilitation specialists embodied in the belief that 'we are all spectators' (in the recovery process). When the predicted outcomes were not favourable, they could be catastrophic for young people who were committed to four or five decades of life confined to aged-care institutions.

The consequences for Freeman's life of the concerted attacks he experienced—most commonly taking the form of professional ostracism and physical exclusion from some hospitals—were often severe. Freeman, however, is adamant that the consequences for patients and their families—for example, those directly affected by the closure of the Brain Injury Therapy Centre—were much more so.

The relevance of Freeman's efforts on behalf of people living with severe brain injury can be evaluated much more clearly after an interval of 25 years, in terms of both scientific basis and clinical outcomes. The manner in which recent investigation of brain function following injury has supported his theories about recovery is summarised above together with endorsements, by well-qualified professionals, of the value of clinical outcomes possible with his approach. Recognition of that value has been reflected by the incorporation of many of Freeman's proposals into what is now mainstream practice.

A phenomenon attributable to advances in brain-scanning technology and the consequent recognition that patients who are clinically regarded as unconscious may not necessarily be so has been increasing advocacy for the replacement of the term 'vegetative' with descriptions that are biologically more accurate and less crass. It may be recalled from earlier chapters that many of the patients whom Freeman was asked to examine had been diagnosed as vegetative, which exacerbated family distress.

9. Some conclusions

The history of Ted Freeman's commitment to improving the subsequent lives of young people who had sustained brain injuries, and their families, includes many events that neither he nor they are likely to have foreseen. Those events raised issues with particular relevance to acquired brain injury but also suggested broader questions related to more general aspects of systemic healthcare delivery and to medical practice, and the relevance to it of ethics and research. Whilst all of these topics have been considered in preceding chapters, it may be helpful to assemble some of them here in order to consider briefly their wider implications.

Systemic inadequacy in response to catastrophic disablement

Although this story relates to a single medical practitioner and a few hundred patients, it is extremely relevant not only for a much larger group of practitioners and their patients but also for all Australians as citizens and healthcare consumers. Some important general lessons for the existing Australian healthcare system's approach to severe disability could be learned from the story of Freeman, his patients and their families.

Consider the healthcare system as it currently impacts upon people like Freeman's patients. The Australian Government Productivity Commission has done just that. An inquiry into disability care and support was released in July 2011. The Commission's report summarised the situation in the following terms: 'The current disability support system is underfunded, unfair, fragmented and inefficient.'[1] Not bad for openers from a government commission reviewing a medley of government programs.

The section of the Commission's report dealing with 'catastrophic injury' could easily be read as an account of many of the patients whose stories were told in Chapter 2. The report observes that '[s]evere brain injury and spinal cord injury are the most common types of serious or catastrophic injury'.[2] Expanding on the patient profile, the report concludes that '[t]hese injuries are mostly experienced by young men aged less than 30 years old and usually entail a

---

1   Australian Government Productivity Commission (2011) *Productivity Commission Inquiry Report. Disability Care and Support.* p. 2.
2   Ibid., p. 794.

period of initial acute care and intensive medical and social rehabilitation to return to some level of independence'. It added: 'Around half of all catastrophic injuries are the result of motor vehicle accidents.'[3]

Freeman's concept of the three accidents affecting people with severe brain injury has been described above. He envisaged the 'third accident' as being an exacerbation of pre-existing disability by inappropriate treatment procedures. This issue is picked up in the Report when it argues:

> People with disability and their families often experience severe social, financial and personal disadvantages over their whole life. While some of this is due to the disability in the first place, much is also due to the dysfunctional nature of the 'system' providing them with support.[4]

In a comment that accords all too accurately with Freeman's description of the conditions in which patients were kept in Weemala as 'repulsive', the report discusses 'leaving people in increasingly abhorrent conditions'.

Some general inadequacies of a healthcare system which regularly fails patients undergoing a slow recovery after severe brain injury were identified in the Report. The experiences of Freeman's patients raise concerns about the attitudes and practices of some health professionals towards people with potentially catastrophic levels of disability, including those with other serious physical injuries such as quadriplegia.

Prognostic nihilism becomes self-fulfilling

Freeman's story should direct attention to the entrenched negative attitudes of many of the medical practitioners who were responsible for the early care of those people who later came to Freeman's attention. The family accounts provided in Chapter 3 are representative of the much larger group from which they were drawn. There was no collaboration involved in their writing, yet there are some very consistent features. Apart from the liberal use of the term 'vegetative', the overwhelming impression with which one is left is that of a consistent negativity, often verging on nihilism, on the part of clinicians.

It is both prudent and reasonable for a clinician to be guarded in issuing a prognosis to a family. One might hope that the practitioner keeps two things in mind. The first of these is to provide information that, to the best of his or her ability, is likely to be accurate. The second, surely, is to consider the likely impact of that information on the patient's family and to attempt to present this

---

3   Ibid., p. 793.
4   Ibid., p. 155.

in a manner that will avoid, as much as possible, the aggravation of that grief which has already stricken them. The first can be based on knowledge gleaned from a textbook; the second requires rather more.

Prognostic caution can never provide an excuse for the crass advice to commit a family member to an institution and then forget him or her. Yet this advice recurs too frequently in family accounts of medical interviews to be a quirk of memory on the part of family members. It is not possible after this interval to account adequately for this attitude, but a number of explanations seem possible.

The first is that no practitioner wishes to be proved wrong in issuing a prognosis. An encounter between the acute-care clinician and any of Freeman's patients five years later would have been rare. Given the way in which the system works, it is unlikely that there would have been any awareness (on the part of the acute-care clinician) of whether a patient had confounded a prognosis by attaining some unpredicted level of recovery. A generally applicable message here is surely that any doctor practising in a specialised area who lacks access to long-term information concerning patients encountered only during the acute stage of care makes prognoses at her/his peril.

Nihilistic prognoses have great potential to become self-fulfilling, as exemplified in some of the patient stories in Chapter 2. Freeman was frequently accused of engendering unrealistic hopes, which were most unlikely to be realised, when he suggested to a family that some chance of improvement remained, but surveys of his patients' families, such as those from Macquarie University, and the observations of the social workers participating in the 'Westmead trial' suggest otherwise.

A second possible factor contributing to the generation of predictions of a hopeless outcome in many cases may have reflected the projections onto the patient of a clinician's personal convictions about a patient's feelings. Thus, if *I* would not want to be in *your* situation, then neither should *you*. The fallacy of this attitude has already been discussed. Some may consider a person living with severe disability following a catastrophic brain injury as 'confined to a wheelchair'. Others, including many of the patients, may consider themselves to be 'confined without a wheelchair'. Perhaps more listening to affected families might have served to persuade some clinicians to amend their attitudes and seriously reflect on Freeman's approach. Perhaps not, given frequent medical prejudice against layperson involvement in the rehabilitation process.

Evidence-based medicine in relation to brain injury

Another question exemplified by Freeman's story concerns how one is to test new evidence. The development of evidence-based medicine is ensuring that only therapeutic approaches that are both effective and safe should be promoted. That is a laudable aim; however, it is necessary that the design that is to guide the assessment process in any instance be appropriate to what is under test in that specific situation. The selection by rote of a double-blind randomised control trial to assess the efficacy of coma arousal provides a superb rebuttal of the adage that 'one size fits all'.

A common perception of randomised control trials is that any risk involved in the trial can be expected to impact upon that group of subjects who are allocated to receive the new therapy. This would be envisaged as a positive adverse effect of the new therapy. This concept becomes inoperative when the best available treatment administered to the control group is effectively 'no treatment'. In this situation, the potential risk may be a negative adverse effect on the control group reflecting deprivation of a potentially beneficial therapy. An illuminating slant on the 'orthodox' approach to people remaining in coma (namely, wait and see) was the designation by Chinese researchers of the 'no treatment' approach as 'Western medicine' (Chapter 8).

As designed, the Westmead trial should have been recognised as both unscientific and, even for the 1980s, quite unethical. Some aspects of it raise the question of compatibility between the roles of a medical practitioner *qua* researcher and his or her duty of care as the patient's doctor. This is certainly an issue with much wider and ongoing implications, raising serious questions of real or perceived conflicts of interest. The story of the failed Westmead trial should be recalled in planning any future trial to test new therapeutic approaches that do not lend themselves to the 'standard' methodology.

Another serious concern that emerges from the story of the aborted trial is the absence of any reliable data on the outcomes of the conventional, conservative management of brain injury. The most practical methodology for evaluating Freeman's approach in comparison with the 'best available' alternative would have been to consider his outcomes against those of 'conventional' management. That those practitioners undertaking a conservative management approach were ready to dismiss Freeman's clinical results although they had not been prepared to undertake a formal assessment of the success of their own practices is most revealing. Equally so was the frequent dismissal of his propositions, while ignoring positive clinical outcomes, by decrying the absence of basic scientific evidence to support them.

The closing of the medical mind

One of the most disturbing aspects of Freeman's story is the attitude adopted towards him by some of his professional colleagues. It would be difficult to conceive of a more clear-cut example of closed minds than their repeated refusals to appear on the program of scientific seminars at which he was to speak or to attend meetings of small groups if he was to be present, given that he was an esteemed participant at such events overseas. The general lesson to be learned from this conduct could be that, if one purports to make decisions on the basis of evidence, it is essential that one be open to considering new evidence, even if it is at odds with one's established position.

A few very competent practitioners publicly stated that, whatever the explanation of Freeman's observations, they merited serious consideration. Other colleagues expressed support for Freeman privately but felt unable to acknowledge this to others. The attitude of the second group should raise some questions about the way in which the medical profession conducts itself. It seems probable that at least some of his critics conflated a lack of evidence for any existing mechanism for brain repair with evidence for the lack of such mechanisms. In the same period, there was a complete paucity of scientific evidence underpinning the generally accepted theory—namely, that neuronal repair was impossible, irrespective of circumstances. In recent years, evidence against the conservative practice of management of brain injury has steadily increased. Whereas Freeman's reference to 'plasticity' (a term he was using in the early 1980s) was invoked in the Cuff Report to disparage his approach, the phenomenon of neuroplasticity—that is, the capacity for brain repair—has now been accepted unequivocally

Science catches up with clinical observation

Freeman encountered disbelief when he postulated, on the basis of his observations of recovery by patients with brain injury, that the brain had an inherent plasticity that could provide a basis for recovery. Two decades on, the adult human brain is known to possess stem cells able to give rise to new neurons. The concept of plasticity is accepted by all! Nevertheless, one should now be cautious in automatically attributing recovery from brain injury exclusively to the generation of new neurons.

Much of the disability associated with traumatic brain injury may reflect interruption of pathways between neurons. Plasticity may depend on partial reconstitution of these, or the recruitment of alternative, undamaged pathways, as much as on new cell formation. The acceptance of plasticity by those who previously denied it, explicitly on the basis of the subsequent discovery of new cell generation in the brain, rather than on longstanding clinical observations of recovery, is logically tenuous reasoning. To maintain that brain repair can be accepted now *because* new neurons can be formed may be as wide of the mark as was the previous dogma, which held that repair was precluded *because* they would not.

Australian isolation

Other very serious questions that are raised by the Freeman experience concern the manner in which changes in clinical practice become accepted or are rejected and the value of empirical evidence in influencing practice. Is it reasonable that medical practitioners are able to ostracise, on the basis of inaccurate claims, colleagues perceived as deviating from accepted practice? Perhaps the most disturbing aspect of Freeman's story is the way in which many Australian practitioners were able to ignore the accumulating overseas evidence pointing to the scientific credibility of his ideas. Given the international acclaim accorded his achievements during the 1990s, the general failure of those Australian specialists responsible for the management of brain injury to acknowledge that reality becomes especially concerning. Inevitably, the question arises as to whether the issue of management of acquired brain injury is an isolated example of this insularity.

What about the family?

One final, and very complex, issue arising from Freeman's story is that of the role of family. In the case of brain injury, this role was determined by the family's intimate knowledge of the patient (literally, 'familiarity'), by the patient's ease when with family members in the home environment and by the family's commitment to help. In a more general context, the family role extends far beyond brain injury. Historically, individuals, whether disabled or not, grew up in a family and grew old and died within that family.

As stated in the Introduction, Freeman's aim in recording his experience, which is shared by this author, is primarily to serve as a 'vehicle of disclosure' in order to bring the events that have been described, and their more general implications, to attention. Whilst the preceding paragraphs may have seemed unduly negative insofar as they deal with practices of the medical profession, one would be remiss if this account did not conclude without re-emphasising the significance of families in all that has gone before.

The battle that confronts the family of a person whose rate of recovery excludes them from accessing regular rehabilitation services accords well with the common truism that 'a serious brain injury affects more than one life'. This battle can be aggravated by healthcare systems that are inherently designed to pick winners by selecting for treatment those people who appear to have the best chance of benefiting from what is on offer. Disagreement over responsibility for funding (for example, between jurisdictions or eligibility for insurance compensation) and territorial disputes within a healthcare system can compound the difficulties.

Modern families and their life patterns have become much more complex. Accompanying the changes, the likelihood that one parent, usually the mother, will not be in paid employment prior to the injury to the family member has diminished considerably, with consequent limitation on the ready availability of care for the injured person in the home. This limitation becomes extreme in the case of a single-parent family or on the occasion when the injured member is the principal income earner.

This volume has recounted the stories of some remarkable families who contrived to assemble extraordinary resources to care for their injured member. The volume has not explicitly recounted the extraordinary social and economic stresses that such families are likely to experience. There is a considerable risk that Freeman's demonstration of the overwhelming advantages for the patient with brain injury of domiciliary rehabilitation in comparison with long-term institutionalisation will constitute a de facto release of government funding agencies from their obligations to this group of patients as well as to many others with disability. Recognition of entitlement to a just level of support for people living with disability, of any variety, within the home environment should be accompanied by recognition of the rights of family members providing care, which are likely to be severely constrained by the accompanying commitments. The commonest constraint occurs when a woman's career is suspended to become a full-time carer. Another unfair constraint is that incurred by a younger person whose educational progress may be severely compromised by a commitment to the disabled family member.

The recruitment, by some of the families, of large groups of volunteers to assist with rehabilitation was an outstanding initiative and, at the same time, a great way of enriching the social capital of their communities. As already considered, the cost, in terms of person hours, of implementing slow-stream rehabilitation is outside the budgetary scope of implementation with paid professional staff. That said, the goodwill of volunteers, like the extraordinary sacrifices of families, must not be used as a means to enable governments to avoid provision of the equitable level of support to which severely disabled members of the Australian community are entitled.

Finally, in considering the situation of the families of people undergoing prolonged rehabilitation following brain injury, the predicament of those who have the injury, but not the family, requires consideration. These are categorised in an earlier chapter as an invisible cohort. Almost invariably, they will have been institutionalised and are unlikely to receive any stimulation from visiting relatives. The numerical extent of the cohort remains to be measured but is likely to be considerable. Their rights are similar to those of other members of the community who are more fortunately placed. Solutions are not currently in prospect. If they are to be sought, at least three responses come to mind. Institutions that have not been planned or structured to provide for younger people who may, to varying degrees, be 'locked in' should release these residents to smaller-scale, purpose-built facilities. Funding to support appropriate staffing of these facilities will be required. Initiatives to foster and support voluntary community involvement to provide plentiful social contact for the residents should be implemented. As in many other areas, when the patient cannot come to the community, the community should come to the patient.

www.ingramcontent.com/pod-product-compliance
Lightning Source LLC
Chambersburg PA
CBHW061240270326
41927CB00035B/3448